Primary Care Orthopaedics

Steven Cutts, Alison Edwards and Ryan Prince

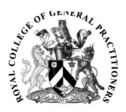

The Royal College of General Practitioners was founded in 1952 with this object:
"To encourage, foster and maintain the highest possible standards in general practice and for that purpose to take or join with others in taking steps consistent with the charitable nature of that object which may assist towards the same."

Among its responsibilities under its Royal Charter the College is entitled to:
"Diffuse information on all matters affecting general practice and issue such publications as may assist the object of the College."

British Library Cataloguing-in-Publication Data
A catalogue record for this book is available from the British Library

Published by the Royal College of General Practitioners 2004
14 Princes Gate
Hyde Park
London
SW7 1PU

Designed and typeset by Discript Ltd, London WC2N 4BN
Printed by The Charlesworth Group
Indexed by Carol Bull

ISBN 0 85084 289 1

Contents

Biography

Steven Cutts was born in Sheffield and initially studied physics at Imperial College, London, and then Medicine at St Thomas' Hospital, London. He qualified in 1992 and is a specialist registrar on the West Midlands Orthopaedics Rotation. He has a long-term career ambition in arthroplasty.

Alison Edwards studied medicine at Oxford and obtained higher surgical training in the West Midlands and Wrightington. In December 2003, she was appointed consultant surgeon at the University Hospitals of Coventry and Warwickshire. She has a special interest in upper limb surgery.

Steven and Alison started writing non-specialist orthopaedics articles for *GP* magazine in 2000 and these articles formed the basis of this book.

Ryan Prince was born in Wales and studied medicine at Birmingham, qualifying in 1995. He became a GP principal in Hampton-in-Arden, Solihull, in 2000, and shortly afterwards was appointed as a lecturer in general practice at the Medical School, University of Warwick. He is also involved in postgraduate medical education as a GP and PCT tutor in Solihull.

Several of our colleagues in the West Midlands also contributed to this text and have since progressed in their careers. Adesegun Abudu is now a consultant at the Royal Orthopaedic Hospital in Birmingham and Darren Clark has been appointed as a consultant in Hereford. Graham Myers is a specialist registrar in orthopaedics in the West Midlands.

Preface

A high proportion of consultations in primary care are of an orthopaedic nature. With an ageing population the emphasis on musculoskeletal complaints looks set to increase. In contrast, orthopaedics does not feature largely in GP vocational training programmes. For this reason, GPs may find themselves falling back on a brief orthopaedic attachment at medical school.

This book seeks to discuss these issues and those orthopaedic problems that are frequently seen by GPs. The text originated from a series of articles written by Steven Cutts and Alison Edwards for the magazine, *GP*. Ryan Prince, a general practitioner, joined the writing team in order to extend the project into a textbook for GPs and to ensure a primary care focus.

We hope that GPs will find this book to be of practical value and a handy reference for future consultations.

Acknowledgements

The authors would like to express their gratitude to Dr Keith Barnard, Medical Editor, *GP* newspaper, and to that publication for permission to reproduce material initially published in *GP*, and to Dr Rodger Charlton FRCGP for his invaluable editorial support and guidance throughout the production of the book.

We would also like to thank Mr M. A. Waldram, Mr Bradish and Mr Glithero for their suggestions on the paediatric and hand chapters; and many other colleagues in the West Midlands for their help and support with this book.

Glossary

ACL	anterior cruciate ligament		IV	intravenous
AP	anteroposterior		MCP	metacarpal phalangeal
APL	abductor pollicis longus		MRI	magnetic resonance imaging
CDH	congenital dislocation of the hip		MTP	metatarso-phalangeal
CMV	cytomegalovirus		MUA	manipulation under anaesthesia
CNS	central nervous system		NHS	National Health Service
CP	cerebral palsy		NICE	National Institute for Clinical Excellence
CPK	creatinine phosphokinase		NSAID	non-steroidal anti-inflammatory drug
CRP	C-reactive protein		OA	osteoarthritis
CT	computerised tomography		PE	pulmonary embolism
CTEV	congenital talipes equino varus		PFJ	patello–femoral joint
CTR	carpal tunnel release		PR	per rectum
CVA	cerebrovascular accident		RA	rheumatoid arthritis
DDH	developmental dysplasia of the hip		RCT	randomised controlled trial
DIP	distal interphalangeal		SLR	straight leg raise
DVT	deep vein thrombosis		SUFE	slipped upper femoral epiphysis
EMG	electromyography		TB	tuberculosis
EPB	extensor pollicis brevis		TED	thrombo-embollism deterrent
ESR	erythrocyte sedimentation rate		TENS	transcutaneous electrical nerve stimulation
FBC	full blood count		THR	total hip replacement
GA	general anaesthetic		TKR	total knee replacement
GU	genito-urinary		URTI	upper respiratory tract infection
HIV	human immunodeficiency virus		USS	ultrasound scan
IHD	ischaemic heart disease		VQ (VP)	ventilation and perfusion
IP	interphalangeal		WBC	white blood cell

In Memoriam
Arthur Conon Stewart
1899–1997

Chapter One

THE ADULT SPINE

Steven Cutts, Adesegun Abudu, and Alison Edwards

Low back pain

Introduction

Low back pain is by far the most common orthopaedic problem in primary care. In 1983, Cypress reported low back pain as being the second most common reason for visiting a physician (the most common being upper respiratory tract infection (URTI)).[1] Low back pain usually reflects minor degenerative changes to the spine and, in modern times, the frequency of consultation has become strongly associated with issues surrounding sickness benefits and litigation.

The number of people complaining of back pain is increasing at an alarming rate,[2] placing an economic burden on society through lost incomes and increased welfare payments.[3] In fact, back pain is now more costly to the UK than any other condition for which economic analysis has been carried out. During the course of the past few decades, it has gradually consumed an increasing share of medical resources. By the late 1990s, back pain was making an unexpected appearance on the political stage.

The Swedish Government became concerned that the number of people off work with back pain would exceed the number of people actually paying taxes within the foreseeable future. A flurry of new 'anti-back pain' legislation soon followed and the number of claimants began to fall. Since then, welfare payments for low back pain have become a significant financial issue in all western countries.

For such a common condition, we know surprisingly little about it. Most of the research concerning back pain has emerged from North America, Scandinavia and Britain. There are so many contributing factors to back pain that it's almost impossible to isolate each potential cause (e.g. smoking, obesity, occupation) and properly assess its significance. Even defining back pain can cause problems. For example, some epidemiological studies require a patient to have suffered from back pain for several weeks in order to be included in a trial whereas others are willing to accept just one day of pain.

Given the widespread nature of simple back pain, it is dangerously easy to overlook the occasional case of sinister pathology (Box 1.1). At the same time, it is unrealistic to investigate every patient presenting to the NHS with back pain. In this chapter we consider both simple back pain and more serious diseases of the spine. The 'red flag' system (Box 1.1) is useful in helping us focus on those patients who require referral and more elaborate investigations.

Epidemiology of low back pain

In modern times, the level of disability associated with back pain has increased more rapidly than with any other illness. During the decade to 1993, outpatient attendances for back pain rose five-fold and the number of lost working days where social security pay was claimed more than doubled.[2] There is no evidence that the prevalence of back pathology is increasing. Instead, the evidence points towards an epidemic of disability associated with simple backache. Powerful social and economic factors are at play here.

Who gets back pain and why?

About 80% of people will get back pain at some time in their lives. In 1992, the annual prevalence rate in the UK was 36%.[4]

The following is true of patients with low back pain:

- 70% describe radiation to their lower limbs
- 40% have symptoms each year or month
- 68–86% recover within four weeks approximately[5]
- 50% of adults seek a consultation
- 10% are seen in a hospital outpatient clinic each year[6] (53% being orthopaedic)
- 5% see an osteopath
- 2% see a chiropractor.

Normally, severe back pain lasts only a few days, although more minor symptoms may persist for many months and most patients will have intermittent recurrence of back pain.[5] Remember that mechanical back pain will tend to be worse with mechanical activity. In contrast, a patient with mechanical back pain can expect relief of symptoms when resting in bed.

Box 1.1   **Common features of back pain and related illness**

Simple back pain
Referral not normally required
- Age at presentation: 20–55 years
- Pain in the lumbosacral area, buttocks, and thighs
- Mechanical pain
- Patient well

Nerve root pain
Specialist referral not generally required within four weeks, provided resolving
- Unilateral leg pain worse than low back pain
- Radiates to foot or toes
- Numbness and paraesthesiae in the same distribution
- Straight leg raise (SLR) reproduces leg pain
- Localised neurological signs

Red flags (signify sinister back pain)
For possible serious spinal pathology prompt referral (less than four weeks)
- Presentation under the age of 20 or onset in those over 55
- Non-mechanical pain
- History of violent trauma
- Thoracic pain
- Past history, malignancy, steroids, HIV
- Unwell, weight loss
- Widespread neurological signs
- Structural deformity

Cauda equina syndrome
Immediate referral
- Sphincter disturbance, sensory level alteration
- Gait disturbance, saddle anaesthesia

Inflammatory disorders
e.g. ankylosing spondylitis (< 1% of back pain patients)
- Gradual onset before the age of 40 years
- Marked morning stiffness, limited range of spinal movements
- Peripheral joint involvement
- Iritis, skin rash (psoriasis), colitis, urethral discharge
- Family history of any particular disorder?

Source: Derived from Royal College of General Practitioners. *Clinical Guidelines for the Management of Acute Low Back Pain*. London: RCGP, 1999.

In the primary care setting, it is simple back pain that predominates:

- <1% of back pain patients have an inflammatory condition
- <5% have genuine nerve root pain
- <1% have serious pathology
- <1% of patients with chronic low back pain benefit from surgery.

However, about 40% of people with back pain worry that their symptoms reflect a serious underlying condition that might affect their employment prospects or long-term health. In most cases, this group of patients is merely seeking reassurance.

People who consult their family doctor with low back pain are also more likely to attend with other complaints. In 1993, Erens and Ghate reported that 53% of new recipients of invalidity benefit described more than one long-term complaint.[7] In particular, it's quite common for several musculoskeletal pains to co-exist in the same patient.[8]

Once a patient is off work with back pain, their chances of going back to work become progressively less with the passage of time. The first 6–12 weeks of unemployment due to back pain are critical, since those who pass through it are at particular risk of never returning to work. Although back pain is usually triggered by a physical problem in the back, psychosocial factors play a large part in determining the speed of recovery.

Pincus et al,[9] writing in *Spine* in 2002, concluded that psychological factors, notably distress, depressive mood, and somatisation, are implicated in the transition to chronic low back pain.

Risk factors for back pain

Age

- Classically, adults in work, 20 to 55 years of age.
- Peak age is 40 years.
- Be wary of back pain in the elderly, adolescent, and paediatric patient.
- Remember that adolescent scoliosis is not normally associated with back pain.
- Over the age of 60, the prevalence of low back pain begins to decline. This reason for this is not clearly understood.

Sex

- Women get back pain slightly more often than men.

- Those experiencing back pain in the late stages of pregnancy are no more likely to be affected by this in the long term than the general population.
- Sciatica is slightly more common in men as is spinal stenosis.

Region/time
- Back pain was just as common in the past. Our response appears to be changing.

Smoking
It is generally accepted that smoking makes back pain worse. However, smoking is so closely related with other confounding factors that its exact role is difficult to determine. Patients for spinal fusion are particularly at risk of non-union, i.e. failure of the procedure, if they smoke.

Obesity
Obesity may not be a great risk factor for back pain. Leboeuf-Yde reported a large meta-analysis of the literature linking body weight to low back pain.[10] He concluded that body weight was a possible *weak* indicator of the risk of low back pain. This and other studies have led some doctors to the counter-intuitive suggestion that obesity has little bearing on back pain. It's actually difficult to know whether an association between obesity and back pain is cause or effect. An out of work, depressed patient with back pain may become less active and eat more. Another part of the problem here is that obesity – like smoking – is such a huge confounding factor that we can't be sure what role it is playing. There are still plenty of reasons to encourage obese patients to lose weight, just as there is ample justification to discourage them from smoking.

Occupation
There's little convincing evidence that a change in employment helps people with simple back pain. Also, in most cases, back pain is probably unlikely to be caused by the patient's job. Some studies suggest that heavy manual workers are slower to return to work than office workers with back pain. However, the same proportion ultimately returns to work in both groups. Disc protrusion has been reported as being more common in office workers than coal miners, although facet joint degeneration is more common in the latter group.

Linton[11] concluded that there is strong evidence that job

satisfaction, monotonous tasks, work relations, demands, stress and perceived ability to work contribute to the likelihood of experiencing future back pain problems.

Litigation

Once back pain is established, the prospect of possible employment compensation becomes hugely influential. Patients may be aware that their back pain represents a route to financial gain and in such cases it can become difficult to differentiate between those who are really symptomatic and those eager to obtain compensation. Always ask a patient what they think caused their back pain and if they are seeking compensation.

The origins of back pain

Of course, low back pain isn't always innocent – like chest pain, back pain may reflect underlying pathology in many organs and structures. We need to be able to distinguish between simple, self-limiting back pain (the vast majority of cases) and other conditions. In this respect, both British and North American guidelines emphasise triage and red flag signs (Box 1.1). It is both impossible and unnecessary to rigorously investigate all patients with back pain; the first priority is triage.

Patients with back pain can be divided into three broad categories:
- *simple back pain* (non-specific low back pain – the vast majority)
- *nerve root pain* (back pain with radiation down the leg below the knee – slipped disc or stenosis)
- *sinister back pain* (rare but important not to miss).

Simple back pain (Box 1.1) may not be associated with any physical signs, although the history may give us some guidance as to the origin of pain.

Facet joint pain classically radiates into the buttock and sometimes down the back of the thigh but not below the knee. On the other hand, pain shooting into the foot is *nerve root pain* and should have a distribution that is at least approximately dermatomal.

The nerve roots are not equally affected. The L5 and S1 roots account for 80% of the nerve roots affected by a slipped or 'protruding' disc. **Sciatica** refers to pain in the distribution of some of the nerve roots that make up the sciatic nerve. Usually just one or two of these roots would be affected.

In **lumbar spinal stenosis**, the spinal canal is too narrow for the lumbar nerve roots and this creates some unusual symptoms. Spinal stenosis is classically associated with pain that is worse when the patient leans backwards. Similarly, leaning forwards or sitting down tends to relieve the pain. Patients sometimes volunteer that they find it easier to walk up hills than down them. Patients with lumbar stenosis often express surprise that they can still ride a bicycle without any trouble. This is because riding a bike involves flexing the spine forwards and when the spine flexes forward, the diameter of the spinal canal increases. Stenosis is discussed in more depth later on in this chapter.

Investigations in low back pain

Simple back pain does not require investigation. A history of recent trauma may justify X-rays to rule out fracture.

X-rays, ESR, and FBC are useful if one suspects sinister pathology. Many patients seem to be greatly reassured by a normal X-ray. As doctors, however, we should be aware of their limitations. Remember that metastatic disease must erode most of the bone before it will be visible on plain X-ray. Older people are quite likely to have evidence of degenerative changes on their lumbar spine X-ray as part of the ageing process. There is a very high false positive rate in lumbar spine X-rays, with poor correlation between symptoms and degenerative changes on the plain film. X-rays are almost useless for detecting a protruding disc. In addition, a lumbar spine X-ray delivers a radiation dose to the patient equivalent to 150 chest X-rays.

Oblique plain X-rays are useful for detecting *spondylolysis*. However, oblique films are not normally indicated in the first instance due to the increased radiation dose this involves. Plain X-ray as a means of pre-employment screening is not indicated, since the correlation between plain X-rays and employment prospects is so poor.[12]

If there are red flags, further investigation such as magnetic resonance imaging (MRI) or bone scan may be indicated *even if plain films are reported as normal*. In fact, MRI has completely revolutionised spinal surgery and actually changed the way spinal surgery is perceived within the orthopaedic profession. Prior to MRI, far more exploratory procedures were performed, often without benefit. In comparison with the past, patients likely to benefit from surgery can now be selected and their operations planned in advance.

The main problems with MRI (other than cost and availability) are the effects of claustrophobia and the magnetic field on patients. They may find the noisy, confined environment intolerable and request to be taken out. Some may sustain serious injury when placed in the magnetic field if they contain metal in their bodies. In such cases, they should all be screened carefully prior to MRI and refused a scan if there is any concern. Sources of metal can include shrapnel, metal clips in the brain, or iron filings trapped in the eye from a career in engineering. Other contraindications include pacemakers and cochlear implants. For these patients a different imaging modality is necessary.

Box 1.2   **Non-organic or behavioural signs ('yellow flags')**

Professor Gordon Waddell, an influential spinal surgeon based in Glasgow, described during the early 1980s various inappropriate or non-organic signs now known as 'Waddell signs'.[13] These are widely discussed in the literature and effectively represent yellow flags.

Whilst no single Waddell sign can confirm non-organic pathology, the observation of several signs in the same patient should make one suspicious. These include pain on axial loading – i.e. vertical pressure on the head, pain on simulated rotation – and non-anatomic sensory loss; e.g. glove and stocking sensory loss.

It is important not to over-interpret Waddell signs. The presence of non-organic signs in themselves is not pathognomonic of malingering. Non-organic signs often co-exist with more objective, organic physical signs and their presence.

It is difficult for a primary care physician to master a subject like back pain enough to make a reasonable judgment on the basis of Waddell or 'inappropriate' signs, but one should be aware that they exist and that attempts to classify inappropriate patient behaviour in back pain have been made.

Degenerative lumbar spondylosis

When patients with low back pain are referred for investigation, plain X-ray often reveals non-specific degenerative changes. This is referred to as **lumbar spondylosis**, which is difficult to treat. There are likely to be innumerable areas of mild wear and tear at many levels in the spine and the relatively crude option of joint replacement is simply impossible. In the past, many spinal surgeons attempted to treat lumbar back pain by fusing the joints in an attempt to abolish pain. Unfortunately, fusing one joint increases the forces on adjacent joints and it is impractical to fuse the entire spine. Many experts now believe that too many spinal fusions were done in the past and it is likely that this procedure will only be performed in very carefully selected patients in the future.

As a rule of thumb, each consecutive spinal procedure has a lower chance of success.

Treatment for low back pain

Simple back pain is a self-limiting condition and this means that almost any treatment will be associated with a degree of success. People with acute low back pain and associated disability usually improve rapidly within weeks, although recurrences are common.[5] Similarly, when a very large number of treatments are routinely used for the same condition, it usually means that none of them work very well. Indeed, when tested by large-scale randomised controlled trials (RCTs), many treatments actually compare poorly with placebo.

Analgesia

In the first instance, paracetamol (1g orally, QDS) should be taken at regular intervals. A second-line drug of choice would be an nonsteroidal anti-inflammatory drug (NSAID). Both classes differ little in their ability to ease back pain and carry the risk of side effects, especially in the elderly. NSAIDs are not as effective for the relief of nerve root pain or stenosis.

Combinations of paracetamol and drugs such as codeine are effective but cause tiredness and constipation.

Muscle relaxants

Benzodiazepines are effective in reducing pain and muscle spasm but are associated with side effects and dependency. It is important not to continue such prescriptions for more than two weeks.

Opiates

These should be avoided as the side effects generally outweigh any benefits.[14]

Antidepressants

Low dose tricyclic antidepressants are often given in the primary care setting. It should be noted that their efficacy in the treatment of acute back pain has not been demonstrated by RCT.

Bed rest

Contrary to traditional belief, RCTs have shown that even two to seven days of bed rest is less effective than placebo. Most authorities agree it's actually better to stay active – bed rest in itself is either of no use or slows recovery.

Return to normal activities

RCTs have shown that an early return to normal activity results in patients using less analgesia and experiencing less disability.

Exercises

Physiotherapy exercises may produce short-term symptomatic improvement in cases of acute low back pain. If a patient hasn't gone back to work after six weeks they should be referred for rehabilitation exercises.

Manipulation

It is a sign of popular dissatisfaction with doctors that so many patients with back pain turn to spinal manipulation by non-doctors. There is modest evidence that manipulation is effective in acute back pain and weaker evidence that it is effective in chronic back pain. In skilled hands it is a low-risk procedure. Shekelle *et al* reported an assessment of the benefits of spinal manipulation in 1992 and found the results inconclusive.[15]

Ice, heat, short wave diathermy, acupuncture, transcutaneous electrical nerve stimulation (TENS), massage, and ultrasound

Although these treatments are very popular and generally harmless, their effectiveness has yet to be established by RCT.

Biofeedback, shoe insoles and shoe lifts, lumbar corsets and supports, ligamentous injections

Again, hard evidence that these are effective in the treatment of acute low back pain is lacking.

Epidural steroid injections

Administration of epidural steroid injections is considered to be worthwhile in cases of low back pain with sciatica, but this option is less effective where there is no radiation of pain.

Facet joint injections

Although commonly performed, hard evidence of relief of back pain is lacking.

Box 1.3   **Back pain treatments to AVOID**
- narcotics for more than two weeks
- benzodiazepines for more than two weeks
- colchicine
- systemic steroids
- bed rest with traction
- manipulation under general anaesthetic (GA)
- plaster jackets

All are either dangerous or ineffective.

Prevention of simple back pain

There is little hard evidence that back pain or disc prolapse can be prevented. Advice on proper manual handling in the workplace and smoking cessation are logical preventative measures.

Secondary prevention. Appropriate management of those already suffering from back pain can be effective.

Tertiary prevention. Rehabilitation to reduce the impact of back pain both socially and professionally. This includes physiotherapy and advice on exercise.

Low back pain in the future

We need to encourage more appropriate referral of back pain problems, since those with simple back pain threaten to overburden NHS resources. This can best be done by heeding the clinical guidelines and following the diagnostic triage.

Sciatica

In sciatica, pain radiates down the length of the leg below the knee and sometimes into the foot and toes. In contrast, low back pain and facet joint pain do not radiate below the knee. Sciatica is rarely due to pressure on the sciatic nerve. Instead, the problem lies with those nerve roots that join together to make up the sciatic nerve; i.e. L4, L5, S1, S2. This is often due to pressure from a bulging or prolapsed intervertebral discs in the lumbar region, although irritation or venous congestion in the exit foramina may also play a role. It is also possible for a disc to protrude in the thoracic region, but this is very rare – accounting for less than 1% of slipped discs. The discs usually move diagonally backwards to irritate the nerve root just as the nerve is about to exit the spinal canal on its way to the leg. Therefore, the disc between L4 and L5 vertebra would put pressure on the L5 nerve root. In fact, L5 is the most commonly affected nerve root in sciatica. Occasionally, a disc moves directly lateral and irritates the higher root; i.e. a direct lateral L4/5 disc would create symptoms in the L4 nerve root.

Sometimes we refer to nerve root dysfunction as radiculopathy. The nerve root about to branch out from the spine is the radical and if this is irritated, the pathology will involve numbness, pain, and weakness in the distribution of that nerve root. Spinal reflexes will also be reduced.

If the disc moves directly backwards, rupturing through the posterior longitudinal ligament, it will create pressure on the roots passing down the spinal canal at that level. For a thoracic or upper lumber disc this would mean the spinal cord itself, although thankfully this is unusual. Patients with active inflammatory changes around the nerve root are said to suffer from **radiculitis**. When the patient coughs or sneezes, a shock wave is propelled down the fluid around the spinal cord and creates symptoms along the leg.

Treatment for sciatica

Since 90% of sciatica cases will resolve within six weeks, few patients are offered surgery without an initial trial of conservative management. Rapidly evolving motor radiculopathy would justify an early operation. Surgery to relieve disc prolapse aims to remove pressure and irritation to the nerve roots. The early results are often spectacular, but surgery is expensive and not without risk and, in addition, the longer-term results may be disappointing. It's worth asking a patient to explain how much of their pain is felt in the legs and how much in their lower back. Generally speaking, a patient reporting all of their pain in their legs is likely to benefit from disc surgery. In contrast, a patient with some sciatica but far more severe pain in their lower back is unlikely to benefit from surgery.

Box 1.4   **Treatment for sciatica**

Open discectomy is performed by an orthopaedic surgeon under GA through a midline incision. This is regarded as the 'gold standard' treatment to which all other active treatments are compared (see Figure 1.1).

Microdiscectomy is essentially the same procedure but requires both an operating microscope and the skills of a specialist spinal surgeon. It produces a smaller scar than the open procedure and is considered by many to allow more rapid mobilisation of the patient.

Chemonucleolysis is a minimally invasive technique. It uses the enzyme, chymopapain, to dissolve disc material. Such techniques can only be performed in specialist centres on carefully selected patients.

Other techniques such as automated **percutaneous discectomy** and **laser discectomy** remain experimental.

Figure 1.1
**Open lumbar
discectomy**

Open lumbar
discectomy is
the gold-
standard
operation for
'slipped discs'.

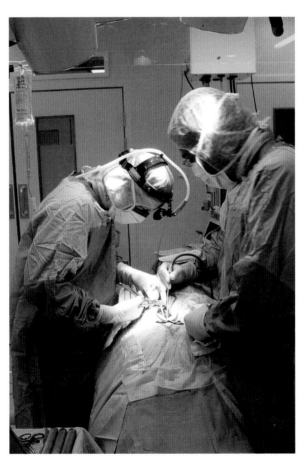

How do sciatica treatments compare?

Approximately 30% of patients treated by chemonucleolysis have disc surgery within two years. Discectomy is significantly more reliable than chemonucleolysis, although chemonucleolysis has been shown to be better than placebo treatments. Discectomy produces a faster return to normal activities. However, the short-term benefits appear to be more obvious than long-term ones. Some studies show no significant difference between those treated surgically and conservatively at the ten-year follow-up stage.[16]

Spinal stenosis

Definition

In some patients the spinal canal becomes too tight for the spinal nerve roots and the nerves begin to malfunction. The problem appears to be more complex than simple mechanical pressure. A reduction of blood flow to the nerves occurs, making the nerve ischaemic and therefore symptomatic. In the long term, mechanical pressure may cause direct injury to the nerve, but this is more of a secondary effect.

Stenosis may be congenital. For example, patients of limited stature with achondroplastia frequently suffer from spinal stenosis. In other patients, the tightness seems to be idiopathic.

In some patients, stenosis appears to be due to degenerative changes in the spine. In others, it is also associated with spondylolisthesis, some metabolic conditions (e.g. Paget's disease), and may be simply post-traumatic. As a group, patients suffering from degenerative spinal stenosis are usually older than those with 'slipped discs'.

In lumbar stenosis, the symptoms often have an insidious onset, although there may be rapid deteriorations. Symptoms are usually precipitated by walking or standing and relieved by rest. As the disease progresses, walking becomes increasingly difficult and the patient begins to stoop. Stooping actually increases the diameter of the tight spinal canal. Patients may find they can walk further by leaning on a shopping trolley. Those who ride bicycles notice that cycling is easier than walking. Walking uphill (where a patient tends to lean forwards towards the slope) is actually easier than walking downhill for patients with this condition.

Neurological examination is often normal in the outpatient clinic. Advanced cases may show numbness or weakness and this is a poor prognostic sign, as recovery of neural function cannot be guaranteed, even with wide surgical decompression.

The main differential diagnosis is vascular claudication. Another possibility is peripheral neuropathy. The following table (Table 1.1) helps us to distinguish between vascular and spinal (neurogenic) claudication.

Table 1.1   **Vascular and neurogenic claudication**

Feature	Vascular claudication	Neurogenic claudication
Pain pattern	Most commonly starts in calves and extends proximally with time	Starts proximally and spreads distally
Precipitating events	Walking	Walking, standing
Relief	Relief rapid with rest, often not required to sit	Needs to sit, takes several minutes
Posture	Normal	Stoops
Exercise ability	Limited range regardless of activity	Can go much further on bike than on foot
Neurological examination	Normal	Frequently normal
Skin condition	Hairless, pale, cold	Normal
Pulses	Reduced	Normal
Past history	ischaemic heart disease (IHD), diabetes, smoking, hypercholesterolemia	Back pain

Investigation

Lumbar canal stenosis is usually a clinical diagnosis. The investigation of choice is an MRI scan. If there's still ambiguity about the diagnosis, nerve conduction studies may help.

Treatment of spinal stenosis

For mild disease, symptomatic treatment only is advisable. More severe symptoms may be temporarily improved by epidural injection, but this will not influence the underlying pathology in most cases, so response is usually limited and brief.

Surgical decompression is an effective method of alleviating symptoms with a relatively good success rate.[17] It is unlikely to reverse objective sensory loss and longstanding motor weakness.

Cauda equina syndrome

Cauda equina syndrome is rare but when it does occur it is a spinal surgical emergency. In this condition there is a sudden increase in pressure on the spinal nerve roots in the lumbar-sacral region and these nerve roots rapidly de-function. If the increased pressure persists for more than a few hours the damage may become irreversible and the patient may be permanently paralysed.

It is important to remember that cauda equina syndrome needs **immediate referral**. Watch out for sphincter disturbance, gait disturbance and saddle anaesthesia. In sudden nerve root compression it may be necessary to do an MRI scan and surgically decompress the cauda equina **within hours**. It is worth knowing your local procedures for accessing urgent assessment for this condition.

If you suspect cauda equina syndrome, do a per rectum (PR) examination. Is there loss of anal sphincter tone? Is there perianal anaesthesia? Offer this information to the on-call surgical team when you make a referral and wish to admit a spinal problem urgently.

Be wary of more modest change in bowel or urinary habit, for example, elderly patients taking painkillers such as codydramol may complain of constipation. In addition, a full rectum will press on the prostate and interfere with urinary stream. Check for this at PR. Check for a longstanding history of gynaecological-related bladder problems in female patients. However, that is not to say that cauda equina syndrome cannot co-exist with the above.

Spinal infection

The incidence of spinal infection is increasing due to higher levels of immigration, HIV, and the resurgence of tuberculosis (TB) in inner city areas.[18] As with all forms of infection, the risk of developing spinal osteomyelitis is increased in the immunocompromised. The infection may be in the vertebrae or involve the disc (spondylodiscitis).

Presentation

Spinal infection may occur in any age group. Children and adolescents are at risk of spondylodiscitis. Above the age of 50 the risk rises again. The causative organism is *Staphylococcus aureus* in the majority of cases, but gram-negative bacterial infections are increasing in frequency, especially amongst intravenous drug misusers. Haematogenous spread is the most common route. The avascular disc is rapidly destroyed by infection, which then spreads to the adjacent vertebral body. TB is a special case of spinal infection – the spine is the commonest extrapulmonary site for TB.

History in spinal infection

Half of spinal infections appear in the lumbar spine. Pain is the most common complaint; over 90% present with back pain, and as many as 50% of patients will have had pain for more than three months. Patients may also present with atypical symptoms such as hip, abdominal, or testicular pain. Constitutional complaints of fever, sweats, and chills may be present in about 50% of patients while 20% of patients will have evidence of neurological involvement on presentation. Any condition that causes immunosuppression increases the risk of spine or disc infection. Approximately 50% of patients will give a history of a preceding infection; e.g. infection of the skin or gastrointestinal tract, or upper respiratory tract infection. Not infrequently, this is a partially treated infection, which will further complicate the treatment of the spine.

Examination

There are often few abnormal physical findings in spinal infection, though the following might be expected in some cases:

- tenderness over the infected vertebrae
- a degree of paraspinal spasm
- a neurological deficit.

Box 1.5   **Laboratory investigations**
- Haematology: full blood count (FBC), erythrocyte sedimentation rate (ESR) – elevation of white blood cell (WBC) count is seen in < 50%, ESR elevated in > 90%
- Biochemistry: C-reactive protein (CRP)
- Microbiology: blood cultures, biopsy samples, and aspirates from operative samples
- Plain X-rays are still used for initial screening. Plain X-rays may show a soft tissue paraspinal mass or bony destruction and disc space loss.

Imaging for spinal infection

Plain X-rays may show destruction of bone or loss of disc height. A para spinal mass may also be visible on plain X-ray. MRI is an excellent investigation for spinal infection. It is sensitive in early spine infections and clearly defines pathology such as abscess formation or cauda equina compression. MRI may also distinguish between an infection and tumour being present. Bone scans are often requested in painful spinal conditions owing to their sensitivity in detecting spinal infection although their use will not yield a specific diagnosis.

Specialist management

If infection is confirmed, refer to a specialist urgently. **Do not start antibiotics until pathogen and sensitivities have been identified.** Percutaneous biopsy is the best method of obtaining good culture

---

Some spinal definitions

Any word that begins with 'spondylo' refers to a condition affecting the spine at any level.

SPONDYLOSIS – refers to a collection of non-specific degenerative changes in the spine that usually occur with age. These include loss of disc height and osteoarthritic-style changes in the facet joints. There is evidence that they may be accelerated by heavy manual labour and some accidents. It usually affects many levels making a simple surgical solution difficult.

SPONDYLOLISTHESIS – refers to when one of the vertebrae actually slips across the vertebra below it. In the lumbar region the upper vertebra usually slips forwards. Patients appear to have an exaggerated concavity in their lumber spine with their abdomens popping forwards. A surprising number of people have mild and asymptomatic spondylolisthesis, although more severe cases can be more serious and require surgery.

Occasionally, X-rays are reported as showing retrolisthesis where the vertebra moves slightly backwards, but this is just a manifestation of the changes in spondylosis and is caused by loss of disc height. It occurs in older people.

SPONDYLOPTOSIS – refers to extreme spondylolisthesis where the vertebrae slips so far that it actually falls off the lower vertebrae!

SPONDYLOLYSIS – is disruption in the pars interarticularis at the back of the vertebra, which is the most common cause of low back pain in teenagers. It also predisposes to a vertebra slipping forwards; i.e. spondylolisthesis.

SPONDYLODISCITIS – is infection within the intervertebral disc.

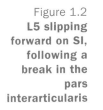

Figure 1.2
**L5 slipping
forward on SI,
following a
break in the
pars
interarticularis**

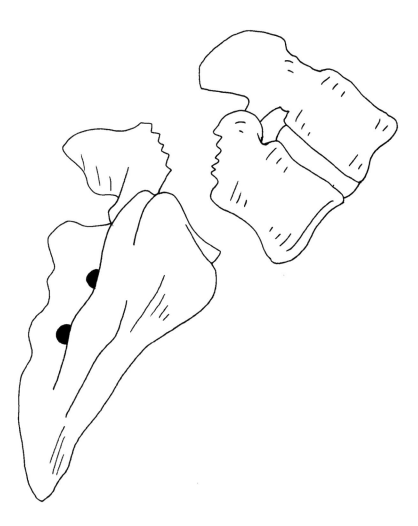

specimens. Appropriate antibiotics can then be given. These may have
to be taken for over six weeks.

References

1. Cypress BK. Characteristics of physician visits for back symptoms: a national per-
    spective. *Am J Pub Health* 1983; **73:** 389–95.
2. Clinical Standards Advisory Group. *The Epidemiology and Cost of Back Pain*. Lon-
    don: HMSO, 1994.
3. Maniadakis N, Gray A. The economic burden of back pain in the UK. *Pain* 2000;
    84: 95–103.
4. Walsh K, Cruddas M, Coggon D. Low back pain in eight areas of Britain. *J Epidemiol
    Comm Health* 1992; **46(3):** 227–30.

5. Pengel LHM, Herbert RD, Mahler CG, Refshauge KM. Acute low back pain: systematic review of its progress. *BMJ* 2003; **327**: 323–25.

6. Croft P, Joseph S, Cosgrove S, *et al. Low Back Pain in the Community and in Hospitals.* [A report to the Clinical Standards Advisory Group of the Department of Health.] Manchester: Arthritis and Rheumatism Council, Epidemiology Research Unit, 1994.

7. Erens B, Ghate D. *Invalidity Benefit: a longitudinal study of new recipients.* [Department of Social Security Research Report No. 20.] London: HMSO, 1993; 1–127.

8. Makela M. *Common Musculo-skeletal Syndromes: prevalence, risk indicators and disability in Finland.* [ML 23] Helsinki: Publications of the Social Insurance Institution, 1993.

9. Pincus T, Burton AK, Vogel S, Field AP. A systematic review of psychological factors as predictors of chronicity/disability in prospective cohorts of low back pain. *Spine* 2002; **27**: E109–20.

10. Leboeuf-Yde C. Body weight and low back pain. A systematic literature review of 56 journal articles reporting on 65 epidemiological studies. *Spine* 2000; **25(2)**: 226–37.

11. Linton SJ. Occupational psychological factors increase the risk of back pain: a systematic review. *J Occupational Rehab* 2001; **11**: 53–66.

12. Ferriman A. Early X-rays for low back pain confers little benefit. *BMJ* 2000; **321(7275)**: 1489.

13. Waddell G, McCulloch JA, Kunnel E, Venner RM. Nonorganic physical signs in low back pain. *Spine* 1980; **5**: 117–25.

14. Bigos SJ, Bowyer OF, Braen GR, *et al.* Acute low back problems in adults. *Clinical practice guideline no 14.* Rockville: US Department of Health and Human Services, Public Health Services, Agency for Health Care Policy and Research, 1994.

15. Shekelle PG, Adams AH, Chassin MR, *et al.* Spinal manipulation for low back pain. *Ann Intern Med* 1992; **117**: 590–8.

16. Weber H. Lumbar disc herniation: a controlled, prospective study with ten years of observation. *Spine* 1983; **8**: 131–40.

17. Turner JA, Ersek M, Herron L, Deyor R. Surgery for lumbar spine stenosis. Attempted meta analysis of the literature. *Spine* 1992; **17(1)**: 1–8.

18. Callister ME, Barringer J, Thanabalasingam S *et al.* Pulmonary tuberculosis among political asylum seekers screened at Heathrow Airport, London, 1995–9. Thorax 2002; **57**: 152–6.

Other sources/recommended reading

Waddell G. *The Back Pain Revolution.* Edinburgh: Churchill Livingstone, 1998. *A highly influential work.*

Royal College of General Practitioners. *Clinical Guidelines for the Management of Acute Low Back Pain.* London: RCGP, 1999.

Gibson JN, Grant IC, Waddell G. The Cochrane review of surgery for lumbar disc prolapse and degenerative lumbar spondylosis. *Spine* 1999; **24**: 1820–32.

A booklet for patients

The Back Book is an evidence-based booklet developed for use with the UK guidelines. London: HMSO, 1996. ISBN 011 702 0788.

Chapter Two

THE HAND

Steven Cutts and Alison Edwards

The assessment of hand problems

A good history of the patient presenting with a hand condition should include age, occupation, the dominant hand, and the functional demands of the patient. The latter is particularly important, because whereas the elderly will often tolerate quite gross hand deformities, a young concert pianist, for example, may require surgical correction for a fairly minor finger abnormality. Remember that signs and symptoms associated with the hands may reflect the presence of systemic disease.

Trigger finger

The cause of trigger finger is not fully understood. Usually a nodule appears in the flexor tendon and as the nodule grows it becomes too large to pass through the A1 pulley in the palm. Eventually, the nodule gets trapped at one side of the pulley with the finger in flexion. Extending a flexed finger becomes difficult, although with enough force the tendon will pop through the pulley as the finger snaps open.

A number of conditions may be associated with trigger finger (see Box 2.1).

Box 2.1 | **Conditions associated with trigger finger**

- diabetes mellitus
- postmenopause
- haemodialysis
- carpal tunnel syndrome
- amyloidosis
- rheumatoid arthritis (RA)
- congenital: usually the thumb, picked up a few months after birth, often bilateral, and said to resolve spontaneously in 30% of cases

Treatment

- *Conservative management*, as the condition may resolve spontaneously. Physiotherapy and steroid with local anaesthetic injection into the tendon sheath around the flexor tendon in the A1 pulley region. A 90% success rate can be expected following two injections.
- *Surgical release* under local anaesthetic, through a 1cm incision. This is very effective. Less than 10% of cases of trigger finger recur after surgery. There is a small risk of adjacent nerve damage resulting in finger numbness. Trigger thumb release carries a higher risk of nerve damage.

Mallet finger

If the extensor tendon is avulsed from the distal phalanx of a finger, the distal interphalangeal joint flops into flexion and the patient cannot actively extend it. The deformity is correctable passively. Such injuries are usually sustained by 'stubbing' the finger. There may be a small avulsion fragment of bone.

Treatment

A plastic splint must be worn for six to eight weeks holding the finger in hyperextension continuously, day and night. (Many patients make the mistake of repeatedly taking them off to see if the finger has healed yet. This tears the tendon apart again.) If done properly, the success rate of a mallet splint is higher than 75%. If there is an associated open wound, surgery is indicated. Surgical options include repairing the tendon or fusion.

Ganglion

A ganglion is the most common swelling in the hand. Ganglia are small lumps, often subcutaneous. Ganglia are harmless but unsightly and often cause pressure symptoms. They are firm, usually non-tender and transilluminate. They are *not* herniations of synovium from the joint! Ganglia reflect cystic degenerative changes within the joint capsule or tendon sheath. They often increase or decrease in size over a period of months.

Common sites for ganglia in the hand

- dorsum of the wrist
- volar surface of the wrist
- flexor sheath of fingers

Sometimes tiny ganglia occur by the distal interphalangeal (DIP) joint of the finger. These 'mucous cysts' are associated with Heberden's nodes and osteoarthritis of the joint. They commonly discharge fluid and may be confused with infection.

Management

- Reassurance: over 40% of cases resolve spontaneously.
- Aspirate the swelling with a wide bore needle under local anaesthetic block. This sometimes works but is associated with recurrence in 50% of cases.
- Surgical excision under regional block or GA. The risk of recurrence is of the order of 5–20%. There is also a risk of damage to cutaneous nerves and numbness around the incision. In the case of DIP joint mucous cysts, fusion of the joint may be recommended where there is significant arthritis and associated pain.

A technique surprisingly well known by patients and their relatives is to hit it with a bible. Of course, any large book would do, as the blow may rupture the capsule and enable the contents to disperse. Unfortunately, recurrence is common with this technique.

De Quervain's tenosynovitis

Some definitions

TENOSYNOVITIS – inflammation of the synovial sheath around a tendon.
TENOVAGINITIS – thickening of the fibrous sheath secondary to inflammation in the synovium.

De Quervain's syndrome represents a tenovaginitis of the first dorsal extensor compartment containing the abductor pollicis longus (APL) and extensor pollicis brevis (EPB) tendons. Clinically, this causes pain at the base of the thumb or distal radius radiating up the forearm that is worse on use. Some authorities maintain that De Quervain's is activity-related. It used to be called 'washer woman's thumb'.

Physical signs: **Finklestein's test** may be exquisitely painful. In this test, the patient is asked to make a fist with the thumb under the fingers and the hand as far radial as possible. The examiner then moves the fist into ulnar deviation. This movement stretches the inflamed tissues causing a sharp and sudden pain.

Treatment

Try conservative measures first – splints, physiotherapy, and a steroid plus local anaesthetic injection into the first extensor compartment. Surgical release is a simple, effective day case procedure. The principal risk is a small numb patch over base of thumb due to damage to a superficial branch of the radial nerve. Although rare, this can be more disabling than the original condition.

Dupuytren's contracture

The exact aetiology of Dupuytren's disease is unknown. Opinion is divided between it being a very slowly growing benign neoplasm or a process of slow scarring. There is laboratory evidence to support both of these views. A common misconception is that Dupuytren's represents an abnormal tendon. This is not the case. The speed of progression is variable, and it is more common in the little and ring fingers. The physical sign that distinguishes Dupuytren's is the nodule in the palm, which may be tender when it first appears.

Figure 2.1
Dupuytren's contracture

This usually affects the little and ring finger.

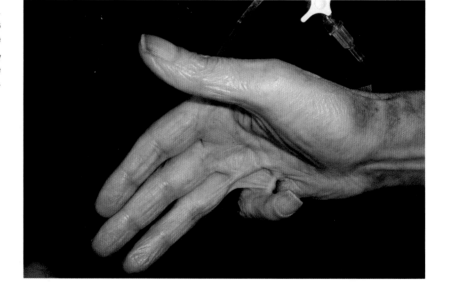

Significant contributory factors

- *Family history*: up to 68% of Dupuytren's patients have a first-degree relative affected.
- *Employment*: many patients believe it is employment-related, for example from using vibrating tools, but it is equally common in left and right hands and there is no medical evidence to support this view.

- *Sex*: Dupuytren's is more common in men, but the disease if present can be particularly aggressive in women.
- *Race*: rare in black, Asian and Chinese communities, more common in people of northern European descent.
- *Age*: occurs in 17% of men over 65 and 30% of men over 85 years of age.

Prevalence depends partly on the threshold chosen for making the diagnosis. A suspicion of Dupuytren's can be seen in the hands of many elderly men. Conversely, younger patients with the condition often have a strong family history, and experience rapid progression and more severe disease. A number of conditions are associated with Dupuytren's (see Box 2.2).

Box 2.2   **Conditions associated with Dupuytren's contracture**
- epilepsy – 42% of epileptics get Dupuytren's, in particular those taking phenytoin
- liver disease and alcoholism
- diabetes
- HIV infection
- smoking
- Lederhose disease, a similar contracture that occurs in the feet
- Peyronie's disease (penile fibrosis)

Surgery for Dupuytren's

Although Dupuytren's won't resolve spontaneously, operating whilst the nodules are still tender may accelerate disease progression. Minor contractures should be left alone unless the patient's occupation demands it.

Surgical options

Correcting the deformity can be attempted by excision or division of the contracted tissue. Proximal interphalangeal flexion is more difficult to correct than metacarpo–phalangeal flexion.

- Surgery can usually be performed as a day case under GA or regional block but sometimes requires an overnight stay.
- Patients should wear a high arm sling postoperatively and begin supervised physiotherapy early to prevent stiffness.
- It can take several weeks for full wound healing.

Risks of surgery

- Incomplete correction.
- Recurrence, either in the same finger or developing in others.
- Damage to the digital nerves. Most of the operating time is spent identifying nerves to avoid cutting them out with the Dupuytren's tissue. Despite such care, temporary finger numbness is very common and permanent numbness results in 0.5% of patients.
- Risk of amputation is rare but obviously serious. Amputation may be necessary in the case of severe deformities.
- These risks are all increased during revision surgery.

Risks of not operating

Once the finger is severely bent into the palm, release may be impossible without vascular compromise. If the skin becomes macerated and cleaning impossible, then amputation may be the only surgical option.

Carpal tunnel syndrome

This is the most common peripheral nerve entrapment neuropathy. The history is classically a middle-aged woman presenting with painful paraesthesiae and/or numbness in the median nerve distribution of the hand, often worse at night. Some patients are vague about the pattern, and may say their whole hand hurts. It is bilateral in 25% of sufferers.

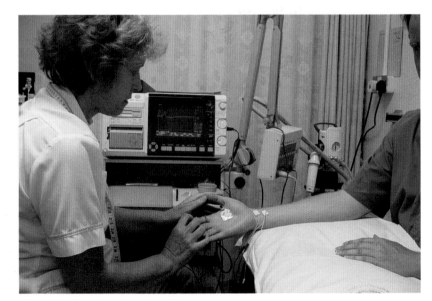

Figure 2.2
Nerve conduction studies to test for carpal tunnel syndrome

These are performed as an outpatient procedure.

Physical signs

- Tinel's sign: tapping the carpal tunnel with one finger creates tingling in the median nerve area.

Figure 2.3
Tinel's test

Tapping the hand directly over the carpal tunnel causes tingling in the median nerve area.

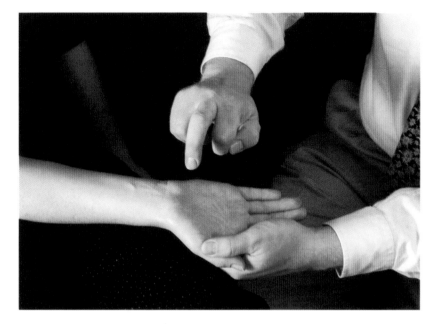

- Phalen's test: full flexion of the wrist for 30–60 seconds re-creates the symptoms.

Figure 2.4
Phalen's test

The examiner holds the patient's arms with both elbows extended and both wrists in maximum flexion. This is a provocative test for carpal tunnel syndrome and it should be carried out for at least 30 seconds. If the patient has a compressed median nerve at the wrist, the test should exacerbate the patient's symptoms.

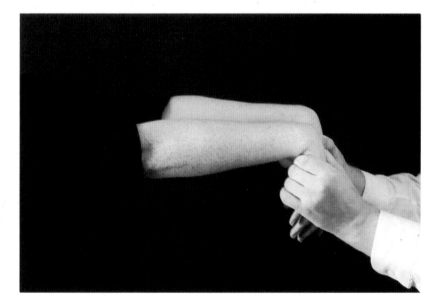

- Carpal tunnel compression test: pressure with the thumb across the carpal tunnel recreates the symptoms.

Figure 2.5
Carpal tunnel compression test

This is a provocative test for carpal tunnel syndrome. The examiner presses down onto the carpal tunnel with his thumb to try to provoke the symptoms of paraesthesia.

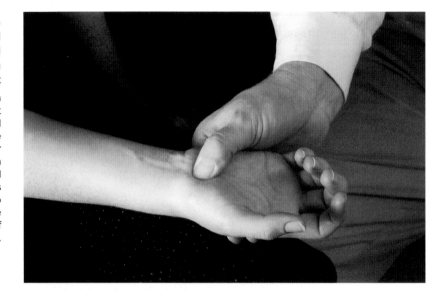

- Wasting of the thenar eminence: often indicates advanced disease.

Figure 2.6
Wasting of the thenar eminence

Compare this dimpled thenar eminence to the convex dome of your own hand. This patient has wasting of the thenar eminence and the problem is much easier to see in profile.

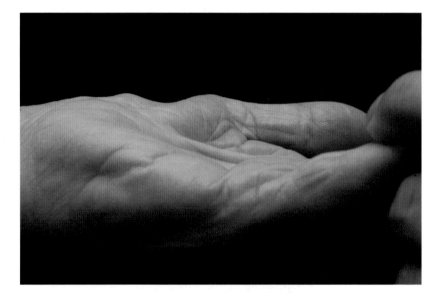

- Check neurology in the arm, because a cervical disc lesion is an obvious differential diagnosis. Also consider thoracic outlet syndrome and shoulder pathology.

Carpal tunnel symptoms may be the presentation of a more serious systemic disease (see Box 2.3).

Box 2.3   **Conditions associated with carpal tunnel syndrome**
- diabetes mellitus
- pregnancy
- menopause
- gout, acromegaly, RA, myxoedema, amyloidosis
- distal radial fracture
- benign tumours
- ganglia in the carpal tunnel

Management plan

Before operating, most surgeons request nerve conduction studies, which improve, but don't perfect, diagnostic accuracy. In some areas patients are referred with a nerve conduction report already organised by the GP. This saves a lot of time, although local protocols may forbid it.

- Conservative measures: Cock-up wrist splints (wrist splint with wrist slightly extended – e.g. Futura splint – may only need to be worn at night); steroid injections around the nerve just proximal to the wrist crease; activity modification.
- Surgery, if symptoms warrant it and compression is confirmed. Carpal tunnel release (CTR) can be performed under local anaesthetic, regional block, or GA, usually as a day case. A greater than 95% success rate should be expected. However, CTR is not as effective if severe long-standing symptoms have permanently damaged the median nerve.

Complications of carpal tunnel release

- Wound tenderness is very common at the proximal end of the wound and may take several months to resolve.
- Recurrence – some have to be re-explored.
- Damage to other structures including branches of the median nerve.
- Operating at the wrong level – nerve conduction studies reduce this risk.

MRI studies show that CTR also tends to decompress the ulnar nerve at the wrist and this may account for those cases where paraesthesiae in the whole hand appears to be relieved by CTR.

Rheumatoid arthritis in the hand

RA is an autoimmune disorder that causes inflammatory changes in many tissues. It is more common in women, although when it does occur in men it can be very aggressive.

- Some rheumatoid patients have no changes in the hands.
- 15% of rheumatoid patients present with signs and symptoms in the hands, classically producing a symmetrical, deforming polyarthropathy.
- Patients mostly complain of pain, deformity, and loss of function.
- X-rays may show periarticular erosions and osteopaenia. The joint space is often preserved.
- Joint and tendon damage can occur secondary to synovitis.
- Ligament erosion results in joint subluxation.

Patients presenting with features of RA in the hand but without an obvious surgical problem should first be referred to a rheumatologist for medical management.

Some hand conditions are more common in RA (see Box 2.4).

Box 2.4   **Common hand conditions in rheumatoid arthritis**
- carpal tunnel syndrome
- Raynaud's phenomenon
- tendon rupture (extensor > flexor)
- trigger finger
- Boutonnière and swan neck deformities
- Cushingoid changes (secondary to steroid therapy)
- De Quervain's tenosynovitis

Rheumatoid deformity

The classic appearance of a rheumatoid hand is a swollen wrist in radial deviation, with a prominent ulna and ulna deviation at the MCP joints – the 'Z' or 'zigzag' pattern. Fingers may show Boutonnière and swan neck deformity.

Surgery for rheumatoid arthritis

There are a number of surgical options for rheumatoid hands (see Box 2.5). The goals of treatment are:

- pain relief

- improved function
- prevention of further deformity
- improved cosmetic appearance.

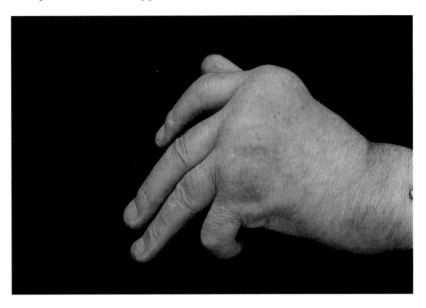

Figure 2.7
Rheumatoid hands

There is characteristic ulnar deviation of the fingers and radial deviation at the wrist. It is believed that the more proximal deformity (the wrist) dictates the more distal (metacarpal phalangeal (MCP) joints of the knuckles). This kind of 'Z' or 'zigzag' pattern deformity is one of the hallmarks of the rheumatoid disease.

Box 2.5 **Operations for rheumatoid hands**

- synovectomy or soft tissue rebalancing
- CTR
- arthrodesis
- arthroplasty (e.g. MCP joint)
- excision of rheumatoid nodules
- tendon repairs or reconstruction

General risk factors

Surgery can be helpful in rheumatoid hands, but it must be remembered that:

- rheumatoid patients have a multi-system illness
- cervical spine changes can make intubation dangerous
- pulmonary fibrosis can also make GA difficult. However, in some cases, hand surgery can be performed under regional block.

Rheumatoid patients tend to suffer from a number of iatrogenic problems. Cushingoid changes from steroids are common, methotrexate causes poor wound healing, and the risk of infection is higher. Good hand function also requires good shoulder and elbow function. When faced with a patient suffering from rheumatoid changes in several joints in an arm, one should usually try to address the more proximal joints first.

Tendon rupture

This is an absolute indication for surgery. Impending rupture often produces pain on use. Extensor tendon rupture is more common than flexor. Early recognition and treatment has the best outcome, but re-rupture is not uncommon.

Metacarpal phalangeal joint arthroplasty

Metacarpal phalangeal joint arthroplasty is a common operation for rheumatoid hands. Once the joint surfaces are denuded of cartilage, pain comes from the joint and not the soft tissues. Swanson silicon rubber flexible implants partly flex and partly act as a piston between the MCP joints. This is a well-established technique, but function may not be fully restored. Despite this, most patients are delighted and cosmesis is much improved.

Surgical synovectomy

From the point of view of an orthopaedic surgeon, rheumatoid arthritis is a disease that causes inflammation in the synovial membrane. All the pain and deformity that follow stem from this initial change. In theory, if one could excise all the synovial membrane, disease progression ought to be halted in that joint.

Not surprisingly, synovectomy has been tested and found to work well for tendon sheaths but not so well for joints. Unfortunately, it is never possible to excise all the synovium. After the operation the synovium regenerates as a normal tissue but quickly regresses to its preoperative level of inflammation. Small joint synovectomy has not been validated by RCT.

It is hoped that, in the future, improved medical treatment for rheumatoid arthritis will make surgery of this kind less necessary.

References

1. Shanker NS, Goring CC. Mallet finger: long term review of 100 cases. *J R Coll Surgeons Edin* 1992; **37(3):** 196–8.
2. Kanaan N, Sawaya RA. Carpal tunnel syndrome: modern diagnostic and management techniques. *Br J Gen Pract* 2001; **51(465):** 311–4.

3. Gerristen AA, Uitdehaag BM, Scholten RJ, *et al*. Systemic review of randomised clinical trials of surgical treatment for carpal tunnel syndrome. *Br J Surgery* 2001; **88(10):** 1285–95.

4. Thurston AJ. Dupuytren's disease. *Br J Bone Joint Surgery* 2003; **85(4):** 469–77.

Chapter Three

TOTAL HIP REPLACEMENT

Steven Cutts and Alison Edwards

Key points

- A successful hip replacement is a life-transforming event.
- Waiting lists for hip replacements are often unacceptably long.
- A painful knee can be misleading when the true pathology may be in the hip.
- The surgeon can have more of an effect on failure rates than the type of prosthesis used.
- Revision surgery should ideally be done in specialised centres.

An overview of hip replacement

Approximately 35,000 primary total hip replacements (THRs) are carried out by the NHS in England every year, and there are about 5000 revision procedures. Unfortunately, the waiting lists for THR within the NHS are often very long.

A successful THR is a truly life-transforming event. One notable feature of the orthopaedic outpatient clinic is the delighted patient. Paradoxically, this has led to unrealistic expectations. Many patients and some doctors have forgotten that THR can be associated with serious complications.

Balancing the risks

All surgery carries risk, including the risk of death. The overall mortality for an adult receiving a THR is probably of the order of 1 in 300. A fatal pulmonary embolism (PE) is believed to occur in about 1 in 600 patients receiving a THR. This figure is perhaps distorted by the fact that so many patients are elderly and have extensive co-morbidity. The mortality for fit young adults is more in the order of 1 in 500–1000. Approximately 1% of patients will suffer from dislocation, although some units are reported to have dislocation rates approaching 5%.

Against these alarming statistics, we must consider the risks of having poor mobility in old age. Patients immobilised by pain are prone to weight gain, depression, an increased risk of deep vein thrombosis (DVT), and chest problems. In turn, obesity carries the risk of diabetes and cardiovascular disease. All of these conditions encourage enthusiastic prescribing by doctors and all carry a significant morbidity and mortality that a THR may help to avoid.

The inpatient stay

A typical inpatient stay is for seven days. The aim is to get patients independently mobile with walking aids when they go home and patients are specifically encouraged and motivated to exercise once they leave hospital, rather than just to rest and recuperate.

Complications of total hip replacement

Infection

Early deep infection is one of the most feared complications of joint replacement surgery. Elaborate precautions are taken by orthopaedic surgeons to minimise the infection risk. Even so, slightly less than 1% of patients develop an early deep-seated infection that will necessitate repeat surgery to remove the prosthesis. The patient will then be left on crutches for several weeks or months whilst the infection is eradicated. Even when another THR is inserted there is still a 10–20% chance of re-infection. The most common organisms responsible are *Staphylococcus epidermidis* and *Staphylococcus aureus*. Risk factors for early infection include diabetes, steroids, being immunocompromised, smoking, and repeat surgery.

Pulmonary embolus

This is believed to be fatal in 1 in 600 THR patients. Most orthopaedic surgeons use some form of prophylactic measure, including warfarin, aspirin, Flowtron boots, thrombo-embollism deterrent (TED) stockings, and heparin. The incidence of symptomatic PE is so low that any trial to determine the relative value of these measures would demand vast numbers of patients. Consequently, there is no real consensus on the best form of thromboembolic prevention.

Recurrent dislocation

This may require revision surgery, which is a longer and more

Figure 3.1
Early deep infection

This picture shows a patient with an infected THR. Less than 1% of THRs become complicated by early deep infection. Next to death, this is the most feared complication of THR.

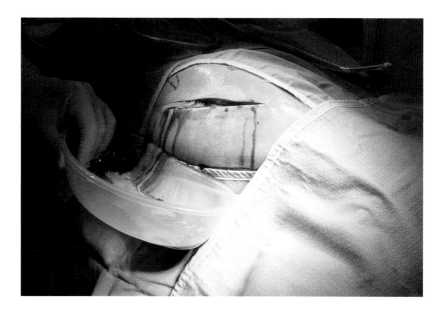

technically demanding procedure. Postoperatively, patients may be required to wear a brace.

Who should perform a THR?

Some orthopaedic surgeons specialise exclusively in arthroplasty surgery. NICE has recommended that a consultant performing hip replacements should perform at least 20 a year. The advent of the consultant who only performs hip replacements may not be desirable, but, equally, THR is not a procedure to be performed occasionally by a surgeon who's main subspecialty interest lies elsewhere.

Key points

- Mortality rate for THR is 1 in 300, but the patients are often elderly and have other medical problems.
- Inpatient stay is about seven days and early independent mobility is encouraged.
- About 1% of patients get post-op infection leading to prosthesis removal.
- PE causes death in 1 in 600 patients and prevention is important.

Dealing with the potential total hip replacement patient

First, we need to assess the degree of disability in relation to the patient's lifestyle. Secondly, we need to try to determine the origin of the pain.

Interpreting the pain

True hip pain is usually perceived in the groin, and often radiates down the thigh towards the knee. More lateral pain with tenderness over the greater trochanter is more likely to be trochanteric bursitis. Pain described as being "at the back of the hip" or "in the buttock" is less likely to be coming from the hip joint, and is probably lumbosacral back pain radiating down to the buttock. Such pain also tends to radiate further down the back of the thigh towards, but not below, the knee. Pain that shoots all the way down to the foot and is worse on coughing or sneezing is more likely to be sciatica. Of course, some patients may suffer all of these conditions at once making it difficult to decide what the real problem is.

The role of hip injections

To try to get round this problem, orthopaedic surgeons sometimes inject the hip with a local anaesthetic and a steroid. This can be done as a day case procedure under X-ray control and does not require general anaesthesia. Occasionally, patients may have a brief exacerbation of their symptoms following injection, but dramatic relief of pain in the first 12 hours suggests the hip is the source of pain. This would favour hip replacement, if the patient's symptoms warrant it. However, if buttock pain persists, this suggests that the hip joint is not the sole source of the pain and that therefore a hip replacement may not eliminate all of the pain.

In some patients a hip injection eliminates pain for several months. This is more often seen in patients with mild to moderate osteoarthritis (OA) or RA where there is a significant inflammatory component. Injecting joints carries a small risk of both steroid-induced necrosis and sepsis. In some very frail and elderly patients pain management is by repeated injections rather than by surgery.

The place of X-rays

Pelvic anteroposterior (AP) X-rays are essential, but the correlation between X-ray findings and pain is often poor. As previously described, hip pain often radiates to the knee. A common pitfall is the patient with the painful knee, where exhaustive examination, investigation and treatment fail to identify or resolve the underlying problem. A combination of hip examination and X-ray may show the true pathology is in the hip joint.

Key points

- True hip pain is usually at the front of the hip.
- Buttock pain is more likely to be referred from the lumbar-sacral spine facet joints.
- Hip injections can aid diagnosis and may give relief for months.
- X-rays are important but do not always correlate well with symptoms.

Who can benefit and which prosthesis?

Indications

Most surgeons would advise trying analgesia, reduced activity, or mobility aids such as a stick in the opposite hand before considering surgery. Pain – in particular night pain – and loss of functional independence are the main indications to perform surgery.

Contraindications

There are surprisingly few contraindications to hip replacement. The main absolute contraindications are active systemic or local infection. Relative indications are gross obesity, and age below 50 years. Obesity makes surgery more technically difficult and increases the risk of complications and early implant failure. Weight loss before surgery should be encouraged.

Choice of prosthesis

NICE issued guidelines on the choice of prosthesis in primary THR in 2000 (see *Further Resources*). It recommend that a cemented, metal-on-plastic primary arthroplasty be used, which has known follow-up data of at least ten years and a revision rate of less that 10%. Over sixty types of prostheses are used in the UK today, but most of these have not been fully validated. Three designs are widely accepted: the Charnley, Exeter, and Stanmore prostheses. All three of these were developed in the UK, and it is worth mentioning that THR is one field in which Britain continues to play a leading role.

Design features

The three designs mentioned above have been around since at least the early 1970s, so there is a substantial body of follow-up data. Charnley's hip prosthesis has a remarkable small head, measuring 22.225mm. This rather odd measurement is a reminder that Charnley designed his hip replacement in imperial measurements; i.e. before we went metric! It's possible that more modern hip replacements are superior to these three but the extensive follow-up data on the classics means we can have a high degree of confidence in the results.

An interesting feature of prosthetic design has been attributed to luck. In the early 1980s, the Exeter group changed the alloy of their hip replacement, so that the surface of the new hip was matt rather than polished. An alarming subsequent rise in failures was traced back to the surface finish, so Exeter now recommends a polished surface.

Follow-up

Sweden's long-standing hip register enables detailed follow-up of all that country's hip replacement patients. This register has demonstrated that failure rates for the same prosthesis can vary by as much as 100% between different surgical units. Clearly, it is not just the prosthesis used, and the operating surgeon still has a major role in success rates. The British Orthopaedic Association began its own National Joint Register in the UK in 2003, with the expectation of better data being obtained from the larger population size.

Key points

- Try simple measures before opting for surgery (e.g. paracetamol, then NSAIDs if they are tolerated).
- There are very few contraindications to hip replacement.
- From over sixty types of prosthesis available, only three are preferred options.
- Failure rates for the same prosthesis can vary by as much as 100% in different surgical units.

Revision surgery and young patients

Revision hip surgery

Revisions are possible when a joint replacement fails, but by the third revision it becomes increasingly difficult. The procedure demands a surgeon who performs a significant number each year, and ideally such cases should be referred to the regional arthroplasty specialist. Not surprisingly, the results of revision surgery are not as good as for primary hip replacement.

Figure 3.2
X-Ray of
Charnley THR

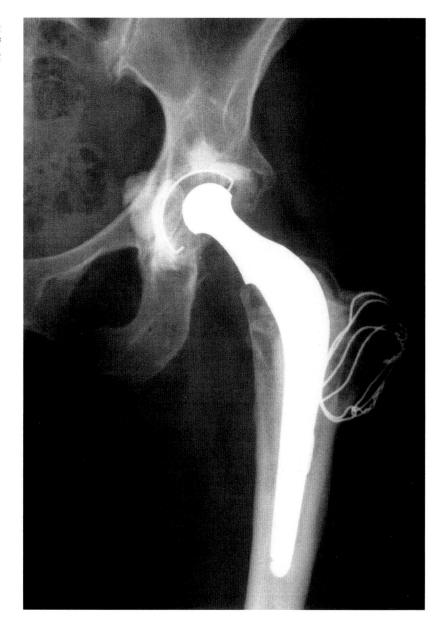

The above picture shows an X-ray of a THR in a fifty-year-old female patient, twenty-five years after her operation. The wires over the greater trochanter reflect a trochanteric approach which was favoured by Charnley himself. The curved metal wire in the socket reveals the plastic socket, which otherwise would not be visible on X-ray. In close inspection, the head has burred a hole upwards into the plastic. Many millions of tiny plastic debris particles will have been scattered throughout this hip joint, although in this case the hip has not become loose. The patient remains asymptomatic and will be followed up in one year.

Most revision surgery for failed replacements is performed following aseptic loosening caused by wear. Wear may occur at any interface, for example bone/cement, cement/prosthesis, or metal/plastic. The debris is not completely benign, as white cells eat the wear particles and trigger a foreign body reaction. At autopsy, plastic particles have been found as far away as the hepatic and para-aortic lymph nodes. The long-term systemic effects of such accumulations are not fully understood.

Trochanteric wires/trochanteric bursitis

Some surgeons approach the hip joint by sawing through the greater trochanter. Charnley himself used this technique, although in modern times it has fallen out of favour in some units. At the end of the operation, the trochanter has to be sewn back on using steel wires. A series of knots are then tied in the wires. Usually this technique is very successful, but sometimes patients come back to the clinic with tenderness over their greater trochanter; i.e. on the lateral aspect of the hip. By pressing one's fingers against the trochanter, the wires may sometimes be felt just under the skin and it is easy to convince oneself that this is the source of the patient's symptoms (this may be impossible in an obese patient). In some cases it is necessary to return to theatre to remove the wires in an attempt to relieve the pain. However, this is not always entirely successful and this problem is part of the reason for a drift away from trochanteric wires. Supporters of the wiring technique point out that a patient may suffer from trochanteric bursitis even if they haven't had a hip replacement. As is often the case in orthopaedics there are several ways of doing an operation and none are perfect.

Total hip replacement in the young

There is a growing demand for hip replacement surgery from much younger patients. In these cases, a specific pathology can usually be identified. The risk factors for early osteoarthritis are shown Box 3.1. Sometimes, the original problem may have been sub-clinical and the patient has no memory of previous symptoms.

The dilemma of the young patient

Younger patients represent a dilemma to the surgeon. A patient in their twenties may well benefit from a THR and be at very low risk of complications. However, the increased demands they place on the hip compared to the elderly and their longer life expectancy make the prospects of revision surgery a virtual certainty.

Box 3.1   **Risk factors for early osteoarthritis**

- SUFE (slipped upper femoral epiphysis)
- Perthes disease
- hip dysplasia
- previous trauma
- congenital dislocation of the hip (CDH/developmental dysplasia of the hip (DDH))
- sickle cell disease
- caisson disease (deep sea divers)
- previous septic arthritis

Whilst simple painkillers and steroid injections into the joint may relieve symptoms for a few years, many of these patients will request surgery at an earlier age than is ideal. Reluctance on the part of the surgeon to operate may be perceived as 'discrimination' by the patient, but there is good reason to try to avoid THR in younger patients if possible. We do know that the younger the patient, the less chance there is that the THR will last ten years. Sometimes, when a young patient receives a primary hip replacement, this is merely the first of a series of hip procedures with an escalating risk of complications.

Hip resurfacing is a newer technology that attempts to address some of these problems. Still in its infancy with respect to long-term outcome studies, and considered experimental, hip resurfacing has

Figure 3.3
Adult hip resurfacing – the face of the future?

Intra-operative picture of completed hip resurfacing.

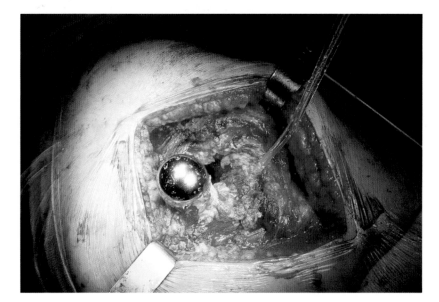

received extensive attention from the media and many patients are aware of it. The current interest in hip resurfacing owes much to the work of Mr Derek McMinn, a specialist in arthroplasty in Birmingham with a long history of technical innovation.

A small (but increasing) number of surgeons have been trained to perform hip resurfacing surgery. Since hip resurfacing does not sacrifice the femoral head, there is potential to convert a resurfaced hip to a conventional THR at a later date. This is seen as one if its main advantages for the young patient.

Figure 3.4
Bilateral hip resurfacing

Compare the size of the metal femoral heads with Figure 3.2. Hip resurfacing creates a normal-sized head and maintains a virgin femoral shaft.

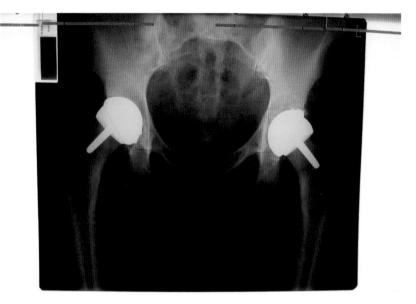

One of the great mysteries of hip replacement surgery is why some hip replacements fail and others seem to continue indefinitely. Until such questions are answered, one should proceed with caution. Some of the younger patients receiving traditional hips such as the Charnley may survive with the same hip replacement for decades, often leading very active lifestyles. Unfortunately, some will always develop complications and require multiple revision procedures. For this reason, a rush to have an operation is not to be encouraged.

Key points

- Revision surgery is needed mainly because of wear and requires expert management.
- Demand from young patients is increasing and specific risk factors are often involved.
- Increased demand and longer life expectancy in the young means revision is inevitable at some stage.
- It is often better to reduce activity than risk surgery too soon.

What does the future hold?

Working on the principle that a hip that erodes less ought to last longer, engineers have designed ceramic heads with super smooth surfaces that, in theory, ought to produce less debris. Whether these have greater longevity in clinical practices will be established with time. Similarly, a case can be made for metal-on-metal prostheses. However, the very tiny metal particles produced from wear represent a tremendous surface area for ion exchange within the body; the long-term implications of this are not yet understood.

Latest developments

New types of prostheses involving materials that allow bony in-growth and more stable fixation are constantly under development. The US is moving away from cemented prosthesis and towards components that integrate into bone. In the UK, NICE has suggested that use of these prostheses should be confined to adequately designed prospective clinical trials until their benefits are proven. The hip resurfacing prosthesis that has been widely publicised in the press is a separate technology and NICE has subjected this to separate recommendations.

Key points

- In theory new surfaces should reduce wear.
- The long-term implications of ingested wear particles are not known.
- Materials allowing bony in-growth are being developed.
- NICE recommends that new prostheses are not widely used until their benefits are proven in prospective trials.

References

1. Williams O, Fitzpatrick R, Hajal S, *et al.* Mortality, morbidity and one-year outcomes of primary elective total hip arthroplasty. *J Arthroplasty* 2002; **17(2):** 165–71.

2. Schulte KR, Callaghan JJ, Kelly SS, Johnston RC. The outcome of Charnley total hip arthroplasty with cement after a minimum twenty-year follow-up. The results of one surgeon. *J Bone Joint Surg Am* 1993; **75A:** 961–75.

3. McMinn DJ. Development of metal/Metal hip resurfacing. *Hip International* 2003; **13 (S2):** 1120–7000.

Further resources

Useful websites

Arthritis Care Organisation: www.arthritiscare.org.uk.

Patient guide to total hip replacement: www.healthpages.org/AHP/LIBRARY/HLTHTOP/THR/INDEX.HTM.

American Academy of Orthopaedic Surgeons: www.aaos.org.

National Institute for Clinical Excellence. *Guidance on the Selection of Prostheses for Primary Total Hip Replacement.* London: NICE, 2000 (under revision). www.nice.org.uk/pdf/Guidance_on_the_selection_of_hip_prostheses.pdf

Chapter Four

THE KNEE

Steven Cutts and Alison Edwards

SECTION ONE – THE YOUNG KNEE

Although knee problems are common in all age groups, many conditions tend to be age-specific. For example, whereas older people tend to suffer from degenerative problems, younger adults are more likely to suffer the legacy of acute trauma. Other conditions such as patella maltracking and Osgood–Schlatter's disease are largely specific to teenagers (Table 4.1).

The knee is a complicated joint and it is often difficult identifying the true source of a problem.

Table 4.1   **Common knee problems**

Young patients	Older patients
Patellar maltracking	Osteoarthritis
Meniscal tears	Rheumatoid arthritis
Osgood–Schlatter (adolescents)	Gout
Anterior cruciate ligament (ACL) ruptures	Degenerate meniscal tears
Osteochondritis dissecans	Loose bodies

Physical examination of the knee

Start by watching how the patient walks. The best way to do this is to watch the patient as they walk into the consultation room, as few people can walk in a 'normal' manner when asked to do so.

Next, we should inspect the standing patient. One of the easiest ways to check for abnormality in a knee is to look at the other side and see if there is any difference. It's a good idea to actually have the patient remove their clothing well above their knees. If they try to compromise by rolling up the trousers you can easily miss an effusion or wasting of the quadriceps muscle.

Genu valgum/varum?

Some patients have an obvious deformity, such as a flexion deformity or genu valgum or varum.

A patient with bilateral valgus knees is sometimes described as 'knock-kneed'. Remember that as a patient develops a **valgus** deformity (Figure 4.1a), the foot deviates laterally, whereas in **varus**, the foot moves towards the midline; i.e. the distal part of the limb is more medial if varus (Figure 4.1b). Varus knees sometimes produce a 'bow-legged deformity'. Valgus or varus isn't actually a diagnosis; it's a physical sign and may reflect many conditions.

The classic osteoarthritic knee is in varus, whereas the classic rheumatoid knee is in valgus. The best time to notice this is with the patient standing upright with their clothing removed as described above.

After the initial inspection the patient lies on the examination couch. If a patient can perform an SLR lying flat, then their extensor

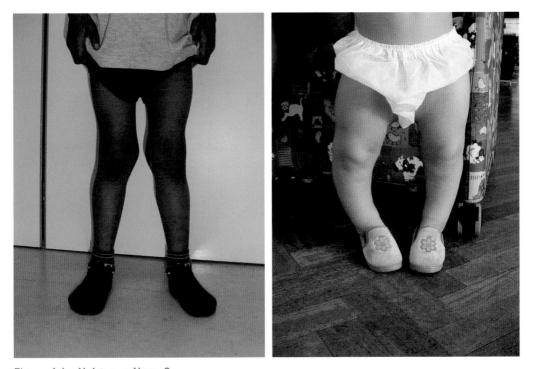

Figure 4.1   **Valgus or Varus?**
Figure 4.1a (left)   **Valgus deformity**
A valgus deformity of the knees in an older child that is already beginning to correct thanks to a stapling operation on the medial side of the growth plates.
Figure 4.1b (right)   **Varus deformity**
A varus deformity of the right knee and tibia in a small child with achondroplasia. The feet are medial to the knees.

Figure 4.2
Axial MRI scan of knee showing patella subluxation in a teenage girl

The patella is well out of the trochlea groove of the femur

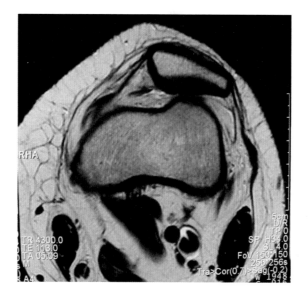

mechanism must be intact; i.e. the femoral nerve, quadriceps muscle, patella, and patella ligament are all in working order.

Next we should check the knees for range of movement. Remember that a healthy young knee should flex until the calf hits the thigh and slightly hyperextends. The active range of movement may be less than the passive range of movement.

Patella apprehension test

If you try to push the patella laterally with the knee slightly flexed, it may be uncomfortable. This usually reflects an unstable patella that is at risk of subluxing or dislocating laterally out of its grove on the femur.

Patella grind test

If we take hold of the patella with a thumb and forefinger and try to rub the back of the patella against the knee, this is a sensitive test for patella–femoral joint arthritis.

Check to see if there is an effusion. If you're not certain that there is an effusion, it's a good idea to try and milk the fluid down into the joint from the suprapatella pouch. This makes the effusion more obvious around the knee cap. If there is a gross effusion then the patella may seem to be lifted away from the knee joint and bobs up and down if you press it into the knee with one finger.

Anterior draw test

In this test, the patient's knees are flexed up to about 90 degrees. If you take hold of the back of the calf with both hands and try to pull the tibia forward and backwards, it may seem to rock a little. This may reflect cruciate ligament laxity or rupture.

With the knee in the same position, most orthopaedic surgeons press their thumbs along the joint line. Joint line tenderness may indicate a tear in the meniscus.

Figure 4.3:
Feeling for medial joint line tenderness

In this picture, the patella has been outlined with a felt-tip pen, as has the medial joint line. Tenderness over the joint line may reflect an injury to the medial meniscus.

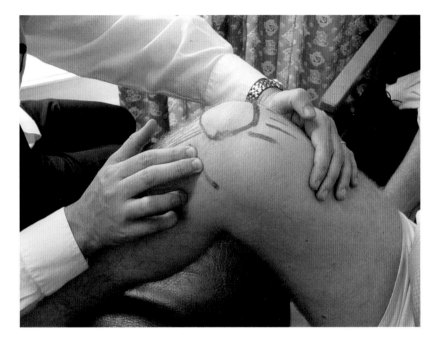

Lachman's test

This is an anterior draw sign carried out at 20 degrees of flexion. The examiner holds the knee in about 20 degrees of flexion and attempts to move the tibia backwards and forwards on the femur. If the cruciate ligaments are intact, they will resist this. If the anterior cruciate is ruptured, there is excessive movement. This is said to be the most sensitive test for cruciate ligament laxity but is difficult in the leg of an obese patient. Subtle abnormalities are easier to interpret if you compare the good side to the bad. Lachman's is probably harder for the non-specialist to master.

McMurray's test

With the patient lying supine the examiner rotates the foot fully outward as the knee is slowly extended. A painful click suggests a tear of the meniscus.

Strictly speaking, the hip should be examined after the knee, as knee symptoms can be referred from the hip.

Biographical note

*Lachman's test is attributed to the twentieth-century American ortho-paedic surgeon **John Lachman** (1956–1989) of Philadelphia. The test was first popularised in the 1970s. It is believed to be the most sensitive test for an ACL injury.*

***Thomas Porter McMurray** (1888–1949) Born in Belfast and worked in Liverpool, initially under the legendary Robert Jones. Later appointed Professor of Orthopaedics in that city.*

Investigations for the knee

Blood tests

If a patient presents with spontaneous swelling, blood tests can help to distinguish simple OA from other pathology. A raised ESR, abnormal RA latex, and autoantibodies may help to identify an inflammatory arthropathy. Urate may be raised in gout (but not always). Blood tests are unlikely to be raised after trauma.

Aspiration

Aspiration of an effusion may be of help, but a patient with an obvious tense effusion would usually need referral to either a rheumatologist or an orthopaedic surgeon. A significant number of patients actually want their doctor to cure their effusion by aspirating it with a needle. Remember, however, that putting a needle into the joint may introduce infection and a chronic effusion is likely to re-establish itself quite quickly.

X-rays

AP and lateral knee X-rays should be requested as weight bearing as some deformities only become apparent when the patient stands up. If the patient describes anterior knee pain you should also request skyline views to demonstrate patella femoral joint pathology.

Box 4.1   **What is an MRI scanner and how does it work?**

In the autumn of 2003, the British scientist Sir Peter Mansfield was jointly awarded the Nobel prize for his work in the development of the MRI scanner.

An MRI scanner is a large, doughnut shaped magnet that the patient has to slide into. The magnetic field inside an MRI scanner is more than 50,000 times as strong as the Earth's magnetic field, although this doesn't appear to present a danger to most patients. The electromagnet provides a continuous magnetic field, day and night, so long as it is maintained at a fantastically low temperature (only a few degrees above absolute zero) by pumping liquid helium around the coil. Unfortunately, this requires a liquid helium pump and refrigeration device to be built next to the scanner. (MRI scanners aren't cheap!) The magnet acts on the hydrogen atoms in water molecules. Every proton in hydrogen is spinning on an axis, just as the planet Earth spins on its own axis, but the direction of the axis is pretty random for every atom. Under the influence of an electromagnet, the protons in water molecules line up, like iron filings under the influence of a bar magnet. Shortly afterwards, the patient is exposed to a radio signal that knocks the spin axes around. When the radio pulse is stopped, the protons attempt to realign again with the magnetic field and in doing so emit radio signals of their own. A radio receiving coil, built around the scanner, picks up this signal and feeds it into a computer that uses it to build up a three-dimensional picture of the proton (i.e. water) density in the patient using a formula developed by the French mathematician, Fourier.

MRI scanning

MRI scanners are expensive to buy (in the order of £1 million each) and expensive to operate, although the unit costs are gradually falling. If MRI scanners ever become cheap and plentiful, they will probably make most other imaging modalities redundant.

Scans may take over 30 minutes and the interior is both cramped and noisy for the patient. A proportion of patients ask to be taken out due to feelings of claustrophobia. Sometimes we can get round this by sedating the patient, although this makes a simple, non-invasive procedure more complicated and potentially dangerous.

An MRI is often performed as a diagnostic aid or to help plan surgery. MRI provides astonishing images of the knee and can accurately diagnose torn ligaments inside the knee. Some units have abandoned plain X-rays and switched to MRI as their first line of investigation. It has even been argued that MRI is cheaper (and certainly safer) than the keyhole operation, arthroscopy. However, the ongoing shortage of MRI scanners means that a more expensive, invasive surgical procedure is often performed.

Unfortunately, MRI remains an expensive investigation and is usually associated with a substantial waiting list. It is also difficult to perform on patients known to have metal embedded in their body (e.g. ex-service men with shrapnel, former machine operators with iron filings in their eyes) as the scanning magnet may tear the metal out. People with pacemakers are also unable to enter an MRI scanner. However, fixed pieces of metal such as a hip replacement are not a problem.

Local protocols may or may not allow GPs to request MRI scans.[2]

It is important to remember that over 85% of knee problems can be diagnosed on the history and examination alone, thus removing the need for more expensive investigation.

Key points

- Simple observation can give useful information.
- AP and lateral knee X-rays with weight bearing can be helpful.
- Blood tests are not helpful in traumatic knee problems.
- Aspiration of an effusion may help diagnosis but consider referral.

Mechanical symptoms in the knee

Locking

True locking occurs when a knee won't fully extend. Remember that a locked knee can still be flexed. If the loss of extension is less than 20 degrees, it can be difficult to detect. It is often useful to make a comparison with the normal knee by holding both legs up by the ankles and watching the knees fall into maximum extension. The healthy young knee will often hyperextend to about five degrees.

In a situation where a patient with a locked knee is anaesthetised for an arthroscopy, the surgeon may notice that the knee has come completely straight before he/she begins to operate. In these cases, the block to extension was pain inhibition. If the problem is a mechanical block – such as a torn meniscus – the knee still will not extend, even when the patient is asleep.

A knee that has 'locked' and then 'unlocked' recently but that is still painful is likely to resolve in a few weeks. As so often in orthopaedics, it is reasonable to manage a locked knee conservatively with a bandage, crutches, and painkillers. After a week or two, the situation may have returned to normal. If it hasn't, we can then consider arthroscopy. A more obvious mechanical block might benefit from earlier investigation.

Patients may also describe episodes of 'locking', 'jamming', or 'sticking', which may resolve by performing a manoeuvre to jiggle the knee out straight. This can be due to a loose body or unstable meniscal tear. The situation can be confused in patients who experience intermittent subluxation of the patella. A persistently locked knee following an injury is likely to need surgery.

Swelling

An effusion is a non-specific but sensitive sign of knee pathology. It usually takes some time for joint fluid to accumulate. However, bleeding into the joint can inflate the knee very rapidly. Injured soccer players may have a knee bloated with blood by the time they've been helped to the edge of the pitch. When you speak to the patient it's important to know how quickly the effusion developed. A patient who develops an effusion within two hours of an acute injury has a 75% chance of an ACL tear and the swelling is largely due to bleeding. Most of the remaining 25% will have a meniscal tear or an intra-articular fracture. If a capsular tear has also occurred, the haemarthrosis or effusion may disperse into the surrounding tissues.

In contrast, delayed swelling that doesn't appear until one to two days after an injury is more likely to be general bruising or a meniscal tear. If you aspirated this swelling with a needle it would be mostly synovial fluid. Swelling usually resolves over the ensuing 2–3 weeks but may recur when the activity is attempted again. If the swelling is only transient and the knee asymptomatic, it may be reasonable to manage the patient in the primary care setting.

Aspirating a knee under aseptic conditions will distinguish a haemarthrosis from a simple effusion. This is often done in A&E. You should collect the aspirated blood in a kidney dish. If there is fat floating on the surface of the aspirated blood then there must also be an intra-articular fracture. If there's no history of injury and the fluid is not bloody, then the fluid can be sent off for analysis. Microscopy, culture, and examination for crystals will help to distinguish inflammatory arthritides.

A hot, red, painful knee with an effusion must have septic arthritis ruled out as a cause and should be referred urgently.

Any skin infection is an absolute contraindication to aspiration because of the risk that the needle may transfer skin bacteria into the knee joint causing septic arthritis.

Giving way

Actual giving way, or a feeling that this might happen, is a common mechanical symptom. Ligamentous instability, an unstable patella, and pain inhibition may cause the knee to suddenly collapse. A feeling of instability on going down stairs, or turning corners, as opposed to pain, may indicate an injury of the ACL.

Pain

The location of knee pain may give a clue to the pathology but is not particularly reliable. Pain at rest or at night may indicate an inflammatory cause. Pain going up and down stairs is often patella–femoral in origin.

Key points

- A persistently locking knee following injury is likely to need surgery.
- An effusion is a sensitive sign for the presence of pathology.
- Do not aspirate in the presence of skin infection.
- Giving way or the feeling this may happen is a common mechanical symptom.

Anterior knee pain

Anterior knee pain refers to a collection of problems at the front of the knee. It is probably the most common problem in primary care in the younger knee. Patients describe pain in the front of the knee or deep in the knee and will often place the palm of their hand over the kneecap when describing it. The pain of patello–femoral joint (PFJ) pathology is worse when going up or down stairs.

Nature has ensured that the articular cartilage on the back of the patella is the thickest in the human body. This is because huge forces (up to six times body weight) are transmitted across the PFJ, especially during squatting. Trying to stand from a low-seated position such as a car chair (especially a sports car) is particularly painful with a PFJ problem.

Symptoms and signs of patello–femoral joint problems

In the young, PFJ symptoms may be caused by malalignment, muscular imbalance, or overuse. Previous patella fracture or dislocation predisposes to PFJ degeneration. Patients who play sports with patellar tendon pain or pain at the inferior pole of the patella may have overuse tendinitis.

Skyline views on X-ray may show PFJ degeneration, tilt, or overhang, but maltracking may not be demonstrated on still images. Even patients with severe symptoms may have apparently normal X-rays. **Chondromalacia patellae** refers to patients with demonstrated chondral degeneration.

Treatment for patello–femoral joint problems

Anterior knee pain can be particularly difficult to treat, but 90% should respond to simple measures. Physiotherapy can strengthen the medial part of the quadriceps muscle and help to redress a functional imbalance. Strapping or taping, flexibility exercises, and activity modification are all sensible.

Surgery may be considered in patients who have failed conservative treatment and who are unable to put up with their symptoms. Realignment procedures, proximal and distal, including lateral release, medial advancement, and tibial tuberosity transfer, all have their place. Most surgeons will offer an approximately 70% success rate and patients are warned that some will be worse after the surgery. Rehabilitation following surgery can last for several months.

PFJ problems are difficult to cure and a number of patients who have problems with their PFJ in their youth go on to develop formal arthritis there in later life.

Key points

- Anterior knee pain is often the result of common inherent anatomical factors.
- Swelling is not usually a feature.
- Patients with severe symptoms may have apparently normal X-rays.
- Physiotherapy to improve medial quadriceps function is valuable.

The anterior cruciate ligament

ACL rupture is common in footballers, rugby players, skiers, and netball players. Many sporting professionals are willing to undergo surgery and extensive rehabilitation to return to the game. Patients may often feel or hear a 'pop' or click during the injury and there is almost immediate swelling and inability to continue. The best way to rupture one's ACL is to sustain a twisting injury to a flexed knee – football players spend a lot of time attempting to change direction on a bent knee.

A young footballer typically describes a twisting injury to his knee, getting sudden pain, and the joint swelling. This initial swelling is mostly blood and is often noticed by the player by the time he has been carried off the field.

The chances of an ACL rupture with this history are 75%. Other causes of sudden bleeding include a meniscal tear, an intra-articular fracture, a synovial tear, patella subluxation or dislocation, or rarely, a posterior cruciate ligament tear.

O'Donoghue's triad is the worst-case scenario. The American surgeon, O'Donoghue described this problem in 1955.[3] It includes ACL rupture, medial meniscal tear, and medial collateral ligament rupture.

Treatment of anterior cruciate ligament rupture

Immediately after the injury, aspiration reveals blood, and removing it eases the pain. The presence of fat globules on the surface of the aspirated blood usually indicates an intra-articular fracture. In most cases, the ligament itself tears, but occasionally, the bony insertion point is pulled out, essentially causing a small fracture which in turn releases blood and fat from the marrow. Avulsion of the insertion point is classically a teenage injury and can be easily fixed by reattaching the bone with a screw. Once the acute pain and swelling have resolved, the anterior drawer and Lachman's test are positive.

People vary in their ability to live without an ACL. Some are considerably disabled, yet others, depending on the sport, continue to play professionally. Chronic ACL deficiency predisposes to further knee injuries. About one-third experience no problems of instability and are able to return to their pre-injury sporting activity. A further third experience instability only when attempting to engage in sport and such patients are usually advised either to modify their activity or have ACL reconstruction if they wish to continue with it. A final third experience recurrent episodes of giving way on a day-to-day basis and definitely require ACL reconstruction. In the initial stages patients would usually be offered intensive physiotherapy to condition their hamstrings before any decision regarding surgery is made.

Why some individuals appear to be more disabled by an ACL tear than others isn't clear. ACL repair has been shown to improve propio-ception[1] in the knee, suggesting that the ligament has a function that goes beyond simple mechanical stability.

Reconstructing the anterior cruciate ligament

Early attempts to reconstruct the ACL used synthetic materials to replace the ligament. This has been abandoned in favour of human tissue, usually autogenous hamstring tendons or a bone-patellar ten-don-bone graft. The procedure requires a surgeon with specific exper-tise in ACL reconstruction and can be performed arthroscopically or by open surgery. Patients need to be highly motivated, as the proce-dure must be followed by protracted physiotherapy. Undisciplined and poorly motivated patients are not good candidates. Middle-aged people with a sedentary lifestyle probably do not benefit from ACL reconstruction. At the other extreme, skeletally immature teenagers present their own problems. Specialist results are reproducibly excellent.

Key points

- ACL rupture is common in men and women who play sport.
- A twisted knee followed by sudden pain swelling suggests ACL rupture.
- People vary in their ability to live without an ACL.
- Autogenous human tissue grafting is now the repair method of choice.

Meniscal injuries

More than one-third of meniscal injuries occur as a result of sporting activities, and soccer accounts for about two-thirds of these. The usual mechanism involves a rotational force applied to a flexed knee. Getting out of a car is a not an uncommon cause. As patients get older, degen-erate tears may occur more easily.

Following the initial tear there may be rapid swelling, or it may occur over the course of the next few days. There is also a loss of about 20 degrees of extension. These symptoms may resolve, but sporadic clicking or locking return later. The knee gives way or swells intermit-tently when sport is attempted.

Examination and treatment

There may be little to find on clinical examination, although joint line tenderness is the most sensitive feature. Ideally, an MRI scan should be arranged before performing surgery.

Surgery to the menisci has a chequered history. It used to be standard practice to completely remove a torn meniscus. Recently, this view has been reversed. The menisci are known to play an important function in distributing body weight across the articular cartilage and their premature removal can precipitate joint degeneration. Many of the younger patients requiring total knee replacements (TKRs) turn out to have had previous meniscal tears. Current treatment is to resect small flaps of menisci and repair larger peripheral tears or detachments.[4] This is to preserve as much meniscus as possible in the hope that in years to come the knee will not rapidly degenerate.

When a meniscus is damaged completely beyond repair, some surgeons have even attempted to replace the structure with a *transplant*. This remains an area of controversy.[5]

Key points

- Playing soccer accounts for many meniscal injuries.
- They occur when a rotational force is applied to a flexed knee.
- Joint line tenderness is the most sensitive feature on examination.
- Removal of the entire cartilage is now avoided, as this leads to early joint degeneration.

SECTION 2 – THE AGEING KNEE

Key points

- Osteoarthritis of the knee is common in those with past injury or meniscectomy.
- Arthroscopic debridement and washout may delay the need for joint replacement surgery.
- Replacing damaged cartilage would be a breakthrough but has not yet been reliably achieved.
- Partial and total knee replacements are constantly evolving.
- The main aim of TKR is the abolition of pain.

Of all the joints in the body, the knee is the most commonly affected by OA. The risk increases progressively with advancing age. OA of the knees is particularly common in patients who have had previous injuries to the joint, especially if they had a meniscectomy.

Joint degeneration may present with gradual pain, swelling, a decrease in range of movement, and crepitus. In more severe cases there may be a fixed flexion deformity. Classically, an osteoarthritic knee develops a varus deformity, whereas a rheumatoid knee develops a valgus deformity. (Plain X-rays of the knee should be requested as weight bearing, as this often reveals these deformities.) In time, the pain may awaken the patient from sleep.

Figure 4.4
Surgical exposure of an osteoarthritic knee, ready for knee replacement

The patella has been everted laterally and we can visualise its arthritic surface.

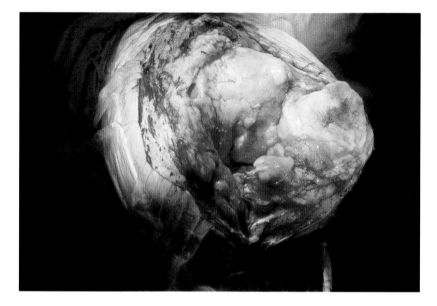

Beware the arthritic hip

Hip pain often radiates to the knee and it is sometimes difficult to be sure what the true source of a patient's knee pain is. For this reason, an examination of the knee is not complete without an examination of the hip. If the hip is arthritic, hip movements may not be painful, but they will have a reduced range of movement. If there is any question of arthritis of the hip, a hip X-ray should be taken. Radiographs of the pelvis often reveal an ipsilateral osteoarthritic hip. When a patient appears to require ipsilateral knee and hip replacements, classic teaching is to replace the hip first, as this may eliminate the knee pain as well.

Conservative management

It is best to begin treatment with conservative measures. Weight loss is known to be effective in knee arthritis. Simple painkillers, walking aids, and activity modification are also eminently sensible. Physiotherapy may help and, in certain circumstances, aspiration of the joint and steroid injections are useful.[1] It's not unreasonable to give an older patient a steroid injection into the knee every six months. In recent years, hyaluronic acid has been promoted as an alternative injection, with the patient receiving a course of knee injections at weekly intervals.[2,3] However, hyaluronic acid injections are expensive and have not yet been fully accepted by the profession.

Glucosamine tablets have also become popular with patients for the treatment of knee arthritis. Supporters of the glucosamine concept argue that it functions as a disease modifying agent, being absorbed into the articular cartilage and subchondral bone. In vitro studies have demonstrated that glucosamine can alter chondrocyte metabolism and this evidence has often been used to justify its use.[4] However, it is difficult to increase the plasma concentration of glucosamine, even by eating huge amounts. In a review article in the *BMJ* published in 2001, Chard and Dieppe[5] accepted that glucosamine was probably safe but pointed out that the evidence to support its use is limited. In a reply, Davide Sonnino pointed out that a failure to modify the disease process in itself is not a reason to stop prescribing a drug.[6] For example, it is routine to give patients NSAIDs as a treatment for OA, even though the drugs are well known to cause adverse side-effects and do not slow down progression of OA.

Glucosamine is in danger of becoming the first agent for which there are more published review articles than there are primary studies. However, Hughes *et al*[7] recently published the results of a randomised trial of glucosamine, suggesting that it was no more effective than placebo. Before encouraging a patient to take regular glucosamine, remember that these over-the-counter tablets are quite expensive. Other recent evidence[8] on the effectiveness of glucosamine has suggested that long-term use could be as effective as NSAIDs for pain relief (NNT5). Glucosamine is now prescribable on the NHS on FP10 prescription.

Whatever else we can say about conservative measures they will always lack the inherent risks of TKR.

Key points

- Joint degeneration presents with pain, swelling, and reduced range of movement.
- Knee pain is often referred from the hip.
- The hip must be examined and, if necessary, X-rayed.
- Conservative measures can be useful before surgical intervention is considered.
- Joint aspiration and steroid injection can give temporary relief.

The role of arthroscopy

There is still considerable debate regarding the value of arthroscopic washout and debridement in the elderly. Many surgeons use these keyhole techniques as holding procedures in an attempt to delay the need for a TKR. Debridement covers procedures such as drilling of bone, shaving loose flaps of cartilage, and chondral abrasion. It was realised as long ago as the 1940s that if a knee was opened and thoroughly washed out, many patients would experience a temporary relief of their symptoms. Unfortunately, recovery was slow due to healing after the open procedure. With the advent of arthroscopic techniques, the procedure has become more popular. General or spinal anaesthesia can be used. By injecting fluid through small portals, an arthroscopic washout procedure can be performed as a day case. The only absolute contraindication is local sepsis.

The results of arthroscopy

Many patients with degenerate knees certainly describe a relief of pain following a knee washout lasting weeks or months. When patients have bone-on-bone articulation with full thickness cartilage loss, arthroscopic procedures have a poorer outcome in terms of pain relief, and they may have no relief after wash out; indeed, sometimes symptoms are worse. In 2002, an influential American study questioned whether arthroscopic wash out was indeed effective.[9] However, the partial relief of chronic mild-to-moderate pain is a notoriously difficult field to work in. There is a powerful placebo component to arthroscopic wash out, but proponents claim that the fluid works by washing out fragments of degenerate cartilage, enzymes, prostaglandins, and small loose bodies.

Other benefits of arthroscopy

Examination of the knee under anaesthesia may clarify fixed deformities or instability. Other damage may be revealed and rough areas of articular cartilage can be shaved. Larger loose bodies can be removed. A symptomatic degenerate meniscus may be shaved back to a clean edge.

Often there is a surprisingly poor correlation between the amount of damage seen through the arthroscope and the patient's symptoms. Some patients present with only recent onset of pain and are discovered on arthroscopy to have significant loss of cartilage. Hyaline articular cartilage in adults is one of those tissues that cannot repair itself after injury. Small defects in the articular surface are often filled by fibrocartilage that functions as a kind of scar. There is some evidence that abrasion to the surrounding articular cartilage during arthroscopy encourages the growth of fibrocartilage.

Key points

- The value of arthroscopic debridement and washout is still debated.
- The only absolute contraindication is sepsis.
- Relief may last for several months, but there is a placebo component.
- Patients' symptoms and arthroscopic appearances do not always correlate well.

Futuristic solutions for the articular cartilage

OA is essentially a disease of the joint surface. Almost the whole of elective orthopaedics focuses on treating this disease but, at present, we have no cure. The implications of being able to replace or renew damaged articular cartilage would be fantastic.

Various methods are on trial. Of these, chondrocyte transplantation has probably received the most publicity. This procedure involves harvesting a patient's cartilage cells and sending them to be cultured in a specialist laboratory. Once sufficient cells have been produced they are implanted in a gel and introduced into the defect under a periosteal seal. They then implant and produce fibrocartilage, which, it is claimed, changes over the course of the next three years into a more hyaline-like configuration. Such procedures have recently been subject to guidelines from NICE. They are not generally available on the NHS. A small number of centres are performing ongoing trials.

Mosaicplasty

Mosaicplasty is another approach to try and deal with chondral defects. This involves harvesting cylindrical osteochondral plugs from a non-weight-bearing area in the knee and implanting them in a mosaic fashion into prepared areas within the defect. The intervening small bare areas fill with fibrocartilage. Some good results have been obtained from this method and a number of surgeons perform this procedure.

Other methods, such as suturing periosteum into the defect, have been tried but are not in widespread use.

Key points

- Various methods of replacing articular cartilage are on trial.
- Chondrocyte transplantation, where cells are harvested, grown in a laboratory, and replaced, has received the most attention.
- Mosaicplasty transfers plugs of cartilage from non-weight-bearing areas to a defect.
- NICE guidelines state that these procedures should not be performed on the NHS except as part of an approved clinical trial.

Partial knee replacement (arthroplasty)[10]

Surprisingly severe deformity can be corrected by knee arthroplasty. Modern knee replacements work well, but the main problem is that many younger patients will outlive their prosthesis. This is not a problem in the elderly. Indications for surgery include symptoms not controlled by conservative measures, worsening deformity, and loss of functional independence. Results are excellent if infection is avoided, but if infection occurs, then multiple operative procedures and severe morbidity may ensue.

The best designs

There are many different designs of partial knee replacements on the market and there is constant evolution of prostheses and of the equipment used to perform the surgery. Degenerate knees are more heterogeneous in their anatomy than degenerate hips, and the variety of types of prosthesis reflect this.

Uni-compartmental replacements

In some patients, only certain parts of the knee joint have been damaged and in these cases, a TKR often seems inappropriate. For this reason, surgeons have developed special prostheses that only replace part of the joint.

Uni-compartmental replacements for the medial, lateral, and, less commonly, the patello–femoral compartments can be performed. Patients must be selected carefully for uni-compartmental replacement. It is technically more difficult to put in than an ordinary TKR, but the inpatient stay is often much less.[11] Some American surgeons are actually performing uni-compartmental knee replacements *as a day case*. Such unseemly haste may reflect the relative youth of the patients and financial pressures as well as the conservative nature of the surgery. If and when a uni-compartmental knee fails, then it can be converted to a conventional TKR.

Tibial osteotomy

In the young patient, a high tibial osteotomy to relieve the load off the main diseased compartment may provide relief of symptoms for some years and postpone a knee replacement. Essentially, tibial osteotomies try to correct deformities around the knee that are probably increasing the load on other areas that may already be damaged. This operation was performed a great deal in the past, but as confidence in TKR has increased, tibial osteotomies have become unusual.

Key points

- Obesity is a disadvantage.
- Results are excellent if infection is avoided.
- Partial replacements with one of many different designs can avoid the need for TKR.
- Fusion of the knee is rarely done but can provide pain relief in patients unsuitable for TKR.

Total knee replacement

TKRs haven't been around for as long as THRs, but they are now very successful. The triumph of a TKR is that it abolishes pain in 95% of patients. The postoperative range of movement is usually similar to that achieved by the patient preoperatively. This means that a patient with a stiff but painless knee is not a good candidate for a TKR.

Development of knee prostheses

Early pioneers of knee replacement used a metal hinge, such as the Stanmore joint. However, this design ignored the complex

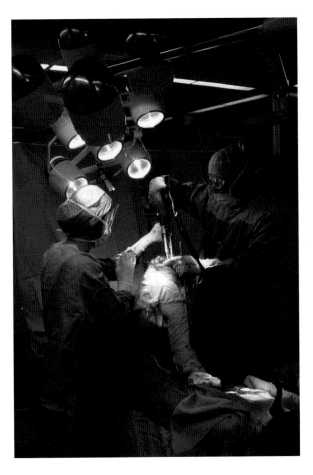

Figure 4.5:
Surgeons
performing
knee
replacement

Preparing the
bones for
insertion of the
components

biomechanics of the real joint, which has rotational and other components. After a few years, many of the hinges loosened and had to be removed. Whilst hinged prostheses are still used under certain circumstances, most modern artificial knees are essentially resurfacing procedures and attempt to replicate the shape and biomechanics of the joint. Whether or not to resurface the patella as part of the procedure is an ongoing area of contention.

How long will a total knee replacement last?

Unfortunately we can never predict how long a knee replacement will last in an individual patient. However, there are some general themes to consider. Generally speaking, high demand users will get fewer years out of their knee. In practice, younger more active patients will walk more miles and live more years than older more sedentary patients and are more likely to outlive their prosthesis and require revision surgery

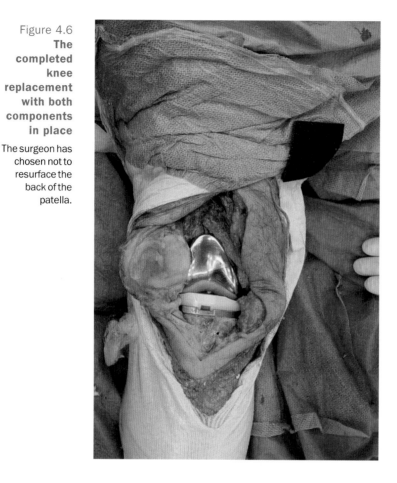

within their own life times. Most ten-year results now show over 90%
survivorship for the prosthesis.[12] Whilst repeated revision procedures
are possible, the risks of each subsequent procedure increase. Each
procedure involves cutting away some good bone and loss of bone
stock is a common fundamental technical problem facing the revision
surgeon.

How successful is a total knee replacement?

Long-term follow-up data are not quite as convincing, but in the me-
dium term, ten-year results of two prostheses, the Kinemax and In-
sall-Burstein knees, show low revision rates.[12] TKR certainly
improves the quality of life for the patient and there's some evidence
that TKR can lead to an improvement in a patient's cardiovascular
health.[13] Patients can expect to regain up to 90 degrees of flexion and
to fully weight bear without pain or walking aids. Overall mortality is

comparable for THR at around 1 in 400, improving to 1 in 1000 for the young. About 1 in 1000 patients are thought to have a fatal PE and most surgeons use some sort of prophylaxis against DVT. Unfortunately, symptomatic PE is so rare that it's difficult to acquire any really convincing data as to which measures best prevent it. The choice of DVT prophylaxis includes postoperative warfarin, aspirin, and TED stockings.

There are risks associated with general or regional anaesthesia, plus damage to neurovascular structures, especially the common peroneal nerve in correcting a valgus knee. It is common for patients to complain of a patch of numbness around the patella where the incision has damaged cutaneous nerves. Other complications include early deep infection, the risk of which is about 1%. This risk is higher in revision surgery and in the immuno-compromised, such as those who have diabetes, RA, and are on steroids. Unfortunately, micro-organisms can live on cement, metal, and plastic and it is almost impossible to eradicate infection from a prosthesis using antibiotics alone. Prosthetic removal followed by insertion of an antibiotic-impregnated cement spacer is usually performed and left for some weeks before second-stage surgery to re-insert a total knee prosthesis is considered. Even then, about 15% of patients will re-infect.

The need for revision

Most revision knee procedures are performed following aseptic loosening and component failure. The patellar component is the most common one to fail. Revision knee procedures are more difficult than primary ones and the results are progressively more disappointing. The big issue is bone stock, as each procedure involves cutting away more bone.

Contraindications to total knee replacement

These are surprisingly few. The patient must be able to do an SLR. Severe neuromuscular dysfunctions militate against success and acute sepsis precludes surgery completely. A neuropathic (Charcot) joint is not suitable for replacement. This is a joint that has been destroyed because the nerve supply to the region has been damaged and the movements have then become totally abnormal; e.g. some diabetics with peripheral neuropathy suffer from neuropathic joints.

Key points

- Despite not being around as long as hip replacement, TKR is an effective treatment.
- The patient becomes pain-free but only retains a similar range of movement to the preoperative state.
- Overall mortality is comparable to THR.
- Average hospital stay is only six days.
- There are surprisingly few contraindications to TKR.

Arthrodesis – fusing the knee joint

Both knee and hip arthrodeses (fusions) used to be common salvage procedures. Although most young orthopaedic surgeons will be unlikely to perform a knee fusion, when all else fails, knee fusion is still performed. The knee is fused in 15 degrees of flexion and the patient has to wear a brace for 12 weeks postoperatively. After this procedure, there will be no joint movement at all, but many patients are grateful for the relief of pain. Occasionally, therefore, this rather drastic procedure is still performed in cases of uncontrolled septic arthritis, complete joint destruction, neuropathic joints, and failed TKRs.

References for Section 1

1. Reider B, Diehl LH, Arcand MA, *et al*. Proprioception of the knee before and after anterior cruciate ligament reconstruction. *Arthroscopy* 2003; **19(1):** 2–12.
2. Watru R, Lloyd DC, Chawdra S. Magnetic resonance imaging of the knee: direct access for general practitioners. *BMJ* 1995; **311:** 1614.
3. O'Donoghue DH. An analysis of end results of surgical treatment of major injuries to the ligaments of the knee. *J Bone Joint Surg Am* 1955; **37-A(1):** 1–13.
4. Boyd KT, Myers PT. Meniscus preservation: rationale, repair, techniques and results. *Knee* 2003; **10(1):** 1–11.
5. Felix NA, Paulus LE. Current status of meniscal transplantation. *Knee* 2003; **10(1):** 13–7.

References for Section 2

1. Raynauld JP, Buckland-Wright C, Ward R, *et al*. Safety and efficacy of long-term intraarticular steroid injections in osteoarthritis of the knee: a randomized, double-blind, placebo-controlled trial. *Arthritis Rheum* 2003; **48(2):** 370–7.
2. Huskisson EC, Donnelly S. Hyaluronic acid in the treatment of osteoarthritis of the knee. *Rheumatology* 1999; **38:** 602–7.
3. Listrar V, Ayral X, Patarnello F, *et al*. Arthroscopic evaluation of potential structure

modifying activity of hyaluronan (Hyalgan) in osteoarthritis of the knee. *Osteoarthritis Cartilage* 1997; **5:** 153–60.

4. Bassleer C, Rovati L, Franchimont P. Stimulation of proteoglycan by glucosamine sulfate in chondrocytes isolated from human osteoarthritic articular cartilage in vivo. *Osteoarthritis Cartilage* 1998; **6:** 427–34.

5. Chard J, Dieppe P. Glucosamine for osteoarthritis: magic, hype, or confusion? It's probably safe-but there's no good evidence that it works. [Editorial] *BMJ* 2001; **322(7300):** 1439–40.

6. Sonnino D. Glucosamine for osteoarthritis. Patients' welfare should be primary concern. [Letter] *BMJ* 2001; **323(7319):** 1003; author reply 1004.

7. Hughes R, Carr A. A randomized double-blind, placebo-controlled trial of glucosamine sulphate as an analgesic in osteoarthritis of the knee. *Rheumatology (Oxford)* 2002; **41(3):** 279–84.

8. Richy F, Bruyere O, Ethgen O, *et al.* Structural and symtomatic efficacy of glucosamine and chondroitin in knee osteoarthritis: a comprehensive meta-analysis. *Arch Intern Med* 2003; **163(13):** 1514–22.

9. Moseley JB, O'Malley K, Petersen NJ, *et al.* A controlled trial of arthroscopic surgery for osteoarthritis of the knee. *New Engl J Med* 2002; **347:** 81–8.

10. Moron CG, Horton TC. Total knee replacement: the joint of the decade. *BMJ* 2000; **320:** 820–25.

11. Beard DJ, Murray DW, Rees JL, *et al.* Accelerated recovery from unicompartmental knee replacements: a feasibility study. *Knee* 2002; **9(3):** 221–4.

12. Scuderi GW, Insall JN, Windsor RE, Moron MC. Survivorship of cemented knee replacements. *JBJS* 1989; **71B:** 798–803.

13. Ries MD, Philbin EF, Groff GD, *et al.* Improvement in cardiovascular function after total knee replacement. *J Bone Joint Surg Am* 1996; **78A:** 1696–701.

Chapter Five

THE PAEDIATRIC HIP

Steven Cutts and Alison Edwards

Key points

- Acutely painful hips in children require urgent investigation.
- When picked up in the first three months of life the prognosis for DDH is good.
- Septic arthritis can destroy a joint in hours – it is a surgical emergency.
- Most children with hip pain have a transient synovitis.

Introduction

The hip joint is crucially important to any child who wishes to walk in later life. One of the great dilemmas of modern orthopaedic surgery is what to do with a patient in their 20s or 30s who clearly requires a THR. Whilst these young adult patients would benefit from such surgery, their activity levels and long life expectancy virtually guarantee that the hip replacement will become loose long before the patient reaches retirement age. It is now believed that many of these patients suffered from diseases of the hip in early childhood. Successful management of these conditions in the young may delay or even remove the need for major reconstructive surgery in adult life. In the future, it is hoped that problems such as DDH will be picked up by universal screening programmes, but it will always be important to remain vigilant in the face of any hip problem in any age group.

Remember that these conditions tend to affect specific age groups. Babies have DDH (formerly known as CDH or congenital dislocation of the hip), teenagers suffer from SUFE, infants are at risk of Perthes', and just about any pre-pubertal child can suffer from irritable hip. Septic arthritis is a rare but potentially devastating disease of the hip. It can occur at any age but tends to be a problem in the very young. Similarly, it's worth noting that CDH/DDH is more common in girls but that most other hip conditions are more common in boys.

Box 5.1   **Main causes of hip pain in childhood**

- transient synovitis
- Perthes' disease
- SUFE
- septic arthritis
- tuberculous hip

Developmental dysplasia of the hip

DDH is a new term that has effectively replaced CDH. This is because the traditional concept of CDH has evolved such that DDH is now a more accurate expression. The new term covers a wide spectrum of features, ranging from a mild abnormality to the frankly dislocated hip. Although this chapter and all recent specialist literature will use the term DDH, the terms CDH and DDH are used interchangeably by many doctors.

An infant with DDH does not suffer from hip pain, although they may well have an abnormal gait. Unfortunately, patients who are affected by DDH in early childhood are at increased risk of suffering from premature hip arthritis in later life. Long-term disability can be avoided by prompt diagnosis and treatment.[1]

Risk factors for developmental dysplasia of the hip

Multiple factors lead to abnormal development of the hip during the perinatal period. The incidence is from one to five cases per 1000 births. It is more common in females than males. The left hip is more commonly affected by DDH than the right. This is because with the head engaged in utero, the left hip levers against the mother's vertebral column. Conditions that tend to squash the baby in utero, such as a first pregnancy or oligohydramnios, predispose to DDH. For this reason, other conditions associated with a tight uterus, such as club foot, may occur with DDH.

In Britain, all babies are clinically examined at birth. Only 50% of children with DDH will have a recognised risk factor. Local screening protocols often screen babies at risk, but it is now known that screening will fail to detect about half the cases.

Diagnosis

Clinical examination alone, including Barlow's and Ortolani's tests (Figure 5.1), will under-diagnose the condition by about 50%. In

DDH, the skin creases may be abnormal around the groin and hip abduction is reduced.

Figure 5.1
**Ortolani's
test**

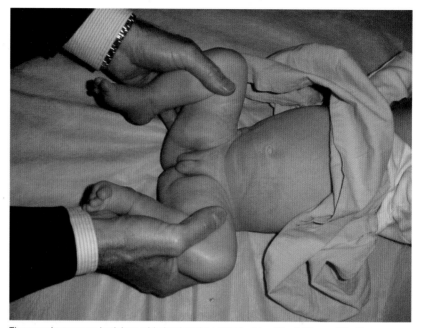

The examiner grasps both legs with the thumbs on the inside of the thighs and the fingers on the outside. Both legs are held flexed at 90 degrees at the hip and abducted together. Ortolani's test detects the 'jerk of re-entry' as a distinct 'clunk' is felt when the hip reduces. This requires the hip to be capable of being both dislocated and relocated. A hip that is permanently dislocated and cannot be pushed back into the socket will not 'clunk'. Often one only feels a clicking sensation, which would warrant being followed by ultrasound.

Ultrasound is now considered the gold standard investigation for diagnosis of DDH. Austria has introduced a universal ultrasound screening programme for all newborn babies. Parents who fail to obtain a 'certificate of scanning' are unable to claim child benefit. A few UK centres now screen all babies at birth and follow up any which may be abnormal. This method has been shown to reduce the late diagnosis of DDH. When picked up within the first three months of life, the prognosis for DDH is good.

Management

The ball of a healthy hip fits the socket exactly. This is because the two components mould around each other during development. Treatment of DDH is based upon keeping the femoral head concentrically located in the socket long enough for normal development to occur. The head is covered more completely by the acetabulum in abduction.

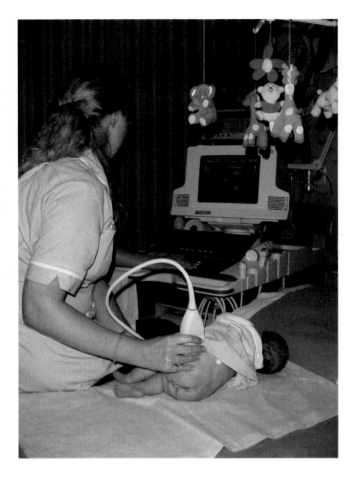

Figure 5.2
Ultrasound scan of the hip

Austria now performs mandatory ultrasound scans on every neonate. Some centres in the UK are also attempting this although, thus far, ultrasound is used in selected cases in most hospitals.

Splinting in a Pavlik harness (see Figure 5.3) will produce a concentric reduction of the femoral head and allow normal development to proceed. A Pavlik harness would typically be worn for between six and twelve weeks. This can lead to a normal hip in over 95% of cases. The later the condition is picked up, the higher the chance of surgical intervention being needed.

Outcomes

As many as 60% of apparently abnormal hips will normalise without treatment after one month and this figure increases to 88% after two months. This leaves one or two patients per 1000 who have a true DDH that will go on to produce pathological changes.

Over time, the untreated hip will develop impediments to reduction. Muscle groups become shortened and contracted, normal acetabular development ceases, and the potential for the acetabulum to resume

Figure 5.3
The Pavlik harness device for DDH

Young children seem to be able to manage quite well in the Pavlik harness for up to three months. The abducted hip is known to be more stable. However, too much abduction can be dangerous and actually cause avascular necrosis.

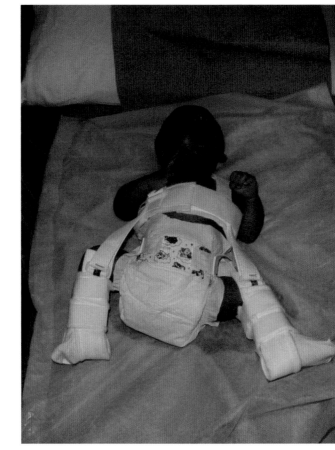

normal growth after reduction is diminished. All this will happen by the age of one year. Persistent severe cases require open reduction and osteotomy (i.e. an operation where the bone is cut with a saw and then realigned). About 2% of cases of DDH are teratological and these are most likely to require surgery.

DDH predisposes to early arthritis. Mildly dysplastic hips may be completely missed and require THR in early adult life. Paradoxically, bilateral DDH is better tolerated than unilateral DDH; patients may have a waddling gait, but at least it is symmetrical and they may function well into middle age.

Key points

Recognised risk factors for DDH are:

- female gender
- breech position, caesarean section, first born
- prematurity, oligohydramnios
- family history of DDH.

Conditions associated with DDH:

- club feet, spina bifida, torticollis, infantile scoliosis
- Down's syndrome.

Clinical examination in DDH:

- Barlow's test – to dislocate a reduced but unstable hip
- Ortolani's test – to relocate a dislocated hip (see Figure 5.1)
- skin creases asymmetrical in the thigh or buttock
- leg length discrepancy
- reduced hip abduction in flexion – should be to 90 degrees
- reduced distance between greater trochanter and anterior superior iliac crest.

Figure 5.4
AP X-ray of the pelvis showing bilateral DDH

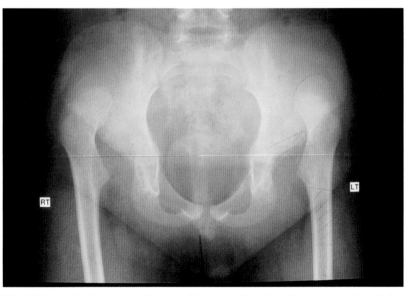

This child was missed at presentation, possibly because the deformity was symmetrical. Both hips are completely dislocated and the sockets are shallow and malformed. The femurs will have to be shortened to reduce the femoral head back into the sockets and pelvic osteotomies will be needed to deepen both sockets.

Transient synovitis – 'irritable hip'

Most children with hip pain and a limp suffer from transient synovitis, or 'irritable hip', a self-limiting condition. It has been suggested that it is either due to a viral infection or an autoimmune process. There is often a history of a preceeding viral URTI or gastrointestinal upset, often involving campylobacter infection. It is twice as common in boys as in girls.

When dealing with what appears to be a case of transient synovitis of the hip, the main anxiety is not to miss the occasional case of full-blown septic arthritis.

Presentation

Pain is usually not severe, but the child may refuse to weight bear on the affected leg. There is usually no pain at rest and passive hip movements are only painful at the extreme range of movement. The child is usually constitutionally well. The ESR is not grossly raised and may be normal.

Management

Septic arthritis is the most important differential diagnosis and investigations are directed to exclude this condition, or fractures around the hip. Once these possibilities are excluded, the management of transient synovitis is rest and appropriate analgesia. If the child can easily weight bear then septic arthritis is unlikely. The child should begin mobilising once the pain has settled. Symptoms resolve within one to two weeks. During the early stages it is important to perform repeat examinations.

Ten per cent of children who have had one episode of transient synovitis will go on to have further episodes. There is no evidence to suggest that there are any long-term sequelae or that hip conditions are more likely in children who have had transient synovitis. In practice most of the young children referred with irritable hip are investigated in hospital to exclude sinister pathology and it's difficult to do this without using simple investigations. In almost all cases, a child who appears to have irritable hip has exactly that. Probably one of the biggest dangers in transient synovitis of the hip is complacency amongst medical staff repeatedly asked to exclude frank sepsis in a patient who turns out to have transient synovitis.

Key points

- Most cases of hip pain in children are due to transient synovitis.
- It is a self-limiting condition, possibly due to viral infection or an autoimmune process.
- The child is otherwise well but will limp.
- There is usually no pain at rest.
- Treatment involves excluding other causes, rest, analgesics and mobilisation.

Septic arthritis of the hip[2]

Septic arthritis of the hip can destroy a joint in a matter of hours. Therefore, sepsis in any joint is a surgical emergency and requires urgent referral. Antibiotics should **not** be started in the community. They will interfere with culture samples taken in hospital and create confusion about the true sensitivities of the organism.

Unfortunately, pus is powerfully chondrolytic, which means that the infection destroys the joint surface. This process progresses rapidly and requires high doses of intravenous antibiotics and open wash out in theatre. The hip, knee, ankle, shoulder, and elbow joints are particularly prone to septic arthritis.

Septic arthritis of the hip usually affects children under two years of age. In full-blown cases, the child is extremely ill and all hip movements are painful. Septic arthritis of the hip is quite unusual in the West; it is far more common in developing countries. Anecdotally, a child with septic arthritis looks ill as you walk into the room. Small children may be irritable at the best of times and septic arthritis of the hip leaves them bed-bound. It's difficult for the child to weight bear through that leg. In short, if you do ever see a case of full-blown septic arthritis of the hip, the diagnosis may not be obvious, but the need for urgent admission will be.

Presentation

Early presenting features in the infant may be non-specific. The hip is held in a flexed, abducted, externally rotated position, and resistance and distress will be noted on attempted movements. There is usually constitutional upset. The older child will be reluctant to weight bear but may localise the pain to the knee. Symptoms overlap considerably with those of transient synovitis but are generally more intense. Pain at rest is a particularly worrying feature. Staphylococcal infection is the most common cause and arrives either from local osteomyelitis or haematogenous spread.

The clinical picture varies with age

Sixty to one-hundred percent of neonates will have adjacent osteomyelitis; this may result from transphyseal blood vessels (which disappear by six months) allowing local spread.

Fifty percent of children aged between six months and two years, with haematogenous osteomyelitis and septic arthritis have evidence of an associated infection. Concomitant meningitis may occur in up to 20% of patients with *Haemophilus influenzae* septic arthritis. However, the incidence of haemophilus is decreasing thanks to vaccination.

Investigations

In full-blown sepsis the child's temperature will be raised and the heart rate increased. Blood tests include FBC, ESR, CRP, and blood cultures. Radiological tests should include plain X-rays, ultrasound and, more rarely, MRI and isotope bone scans.

Treatment

Septic arthritis is a surgical emergency. Most surgeons would take the child to the operating theatre as soon as possible, drain the hip of pus, and further irrigate the joint with saline. An alternative strategy is to try to aspirate the joint using a needle under ultrasound control. If the fluid produced is pus, surgery can then be performed. Antibiotics appropriate for the organism isolated are usually continued for six weeks.

Tuberculous synovitis

Tuberculosis is making a comeback in the West and is more common in families with contacts in Africa and India. The bacillus arrives in the joint by haematogenous spread or from adjacent osteomyelitis.

The disease starts as synovitis and can go on to cause rapid destruction of the femoral head. Healing leaves a fibrous ankylosis with limb shortening and deformity. In the short term, the child requires incision of the infected joint and drainage of the cold abscess, followed by intravenous antibiotics. Ultimately, the patient often requires arthrodesis (i.e. a joint fusion). If the disease has been inactive for many years, THR is an option for adult patients.

Key points

- Septic arthritis is a surgical emergency because it can destroy a joint in a matter of hours.
- GPs should not start antibiotics prior to admission, as they will interfere with blood cultures.
- Pain at rest is a worrying feature.
- Meningitis may occur concomitantly with septic arthritis in a fifth of patients with *H. influenzae* infection.
- Hip aspiration and an arthrotomy are carried out under general anaesthetic.
- Tuberculosis infection of the hip is making a comeback in the West.

Perthes' disease

In 1910, working in three separate countries, Legg, Calve, and Perthes each independently described the same condition in young hips. This remarkable coincidence stems from the fact that X-rays had only just been invented and the beginning of the 20th century was a golden age for original research using X-rays. Some specialist text books still refer to Legg–Calve–Perthes disease, or LCP for short. In everyday conversation it is Perthes' name that is best remembered. Nearly 100 years later, our understanding of the aetiology is still poor.

Perthes' is a self-limiting condition in which the blood supply to the femoral head is cut off and the bone crumbles and dies (i.e. avascular necrosis). The male to female ratio is 4:1, and it typically affects children between five and ten years of age.

In Perthes' disease, the head of the femur experiences a series of ischaemic insults. This is followed by an episode of avascular necrosis, which is, in turn, followed by re-vascularisation and a process of re-modelling. The early, new bone formed has plastic properties although, even after final resolution, the head may well remain an abnormal shape.

Risk factors for Perthes'[3]

- male (80% are boys)
- low birth weight
- low socio-economic status
- passive smoking

In the UK, Perthes' currently affects about 1 in 12,000 children. The

Figure 5.5
AP X-ray of the pelvis showing Perthes' disease

Compare the good (right-sided) femoral head to the abnormal/abducted left side. This particularly spectacular case of Perthes' disease gives the impression of the femoral head being 'bitten off' on the left side.

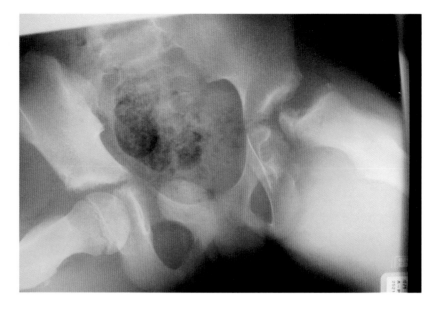

typical age at presentation is between five and ten years. X-rays of the rest of the skeleton often reveal that the bone age is about two years retarded relative to children of the same age. These children may also suffer from short stature, suggesting that Perthes' is part of a polygenetic problem affecting the whole skeleton. More recently, it has been suggested that Perthes' is caused by an abnormality in the clotting cascade.[4]

Perthes' is unilateral in 85% of cases. When it is bilateral, other differentials (e.g. Gaucher's, hypothyroidism, and epiphyseal dysplasia) should be considered. Bilateral cases may be neither symmetrical nor synchronous.

The prospects for recovery are best in young children, who have the most time to remodel. Generally speaking, girls have a worse prognosis than boys. This may reflect the fact that girls stop growing earlier and therefore have less time to remodel. In either sex, presentation above the age of ten carries a particularly poor prognosis.

Presentation

There is gradual onset of pain and the child limps intermittently. The range of movement in the hip is reduced. Unlike irritable hip, Perthes' is persistent. In more advanced cases, the limb may be shorter and both the thigh and buttock on the affected side may be wasted.

X-rays

Initially, X-rays may be normal. Later, they reveal the true extent of the disease. X-rays show flattening of the superolateral epiphysis and later fragmentation.

Treatment

The goals of treatment are to eliminate irritability and to restore and maintain a good range of movement by physiotherapy. For many patients, this in itself may be adequate treatment. More severe cases may require intervention.

Conservative treatment

If the thigh is held in abduction, then the articular surface of the femoral head will be completely covered by the acetabulum. This position of containment is believed to maximise the chances of the successful remodelling producing a spherical femoral head in a congruent joint. Such a position can be held by a broomstick cast applied under anaesthetic and in some cases this process may be assisted by cutting the adductor tendons. The application of a broomstick cast is quite an undertaking for both child and family, and may be in place for a period between 12 and 18 months.

Operative containment

The best way to achieve immediate containment is by performing an operation. This allows an earlier resumption of normal activities than conservative management, although the hip may ultimately have a more limited range of movement. However, this major surgery is usually reserved for older children who have presented late or who have particularly severe problems. As the patient emerges from adolescence, they will probably have a near normal hip, perhaps with slight restriction of movement.

Key points

- The cause of Perthes' is still not clear 91 years after its discovery.
- Presentation is with a limp and pain may be referred to the knee.
- Children under six have a better prognosis.
- Fifty per cent of cases do well without any treatment, but many patients develop degenerative joint disease in later life.

Slipped upper femoral epiphysis[5]

Classically, a SUFE will occur at the onset of puberty in a child who is either very tall and thin or short and obese. The average age at onset is 12 years. It can be confused with irritable hip (transient synovitis).

(NB SUFE is also some times referred to as SCFE; i.e. slipped capital femoral epiphysis.)

Aetiology and risk factors for slipped upper femoral epiphysis

The growth plate represents a structural weak point in the hip and in some children the femoral head appears to slip off the proximal femur. The head itself remains in the acetabulum.

Those most at risk for SUFE include:

- those of Afro-Caribbean descent
- teenagers
- males
- those who are obese
- those with a positive family history.

Twenty-five per cent of cases are bilateral. Bilateral cases are defined as cases where one side occurs within six months of the other. Hormonal changes including hypothyroidism may be implicated. Fifty per cent of cases have a history of injury and 20% of cases have similar slips on the opposite side. There is a risk of osteonecrosis of the femoral head.

History and examination

SUFE can cause hip, thigh, and knee pain. There is often a history of several weeks of vague aching in the groin or thigh in the early stages of the slip.

Examination may reveal that when the hip is actively flexed, it comes up in external rotation. If the slip is significant, the limb may be 1–2cm short. Children may be able to weight bear but with pain. A sudden episode of pain followed by an inability to weight bear usually indicates a more severe slip.

Investigations and treatment

Specialists often perform CT scanning to assess the angle of femoral neck anteversion. If it is less than ten degrees then there is a greater risk of problems.

Most slips are less than 50% and are treated by pinning in situ with

Figure 5.6
**Acute
slipped upper
femoral
epiphysis**

The right hip –
affected by SUFE
– is shortened by
2–3cm and
externally
rotated.
Inserting a pin
into the femoral
head stops the
upper femoral
epiphysis
slipping further
but it does not
correct the
deformity.

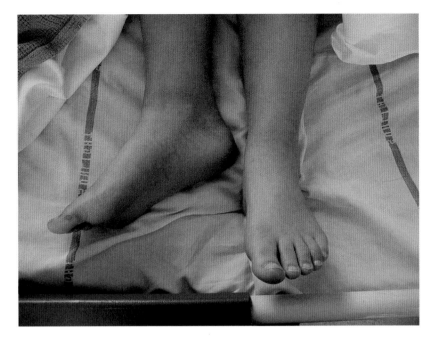

a single screw. A slip greater than 50% requires osteotomy and pinning and has a much greater risk of avascular necrosis. Other complications include limb length discrepancy, gait abnormalities, and chondrolysis.

Longer-term complications include degenerative joint disease, with some former SUFE patients requiring hip replacement in early adult life.

Key points

- Usually occurs at onset of puberty in tall/thin or short/obese children.
- 25% of cases are bilateral and 50% have a history of injury.
- The onset is usually gradual, with increasing thigh, hip, or knee pain.
- An inability to weight bear in SUFE is a bad sign.
- Treatment is with pinning or osteotomy for severe cases.
- Some SUFE patients will require hip replacement in early adult life.

Table 5.1   **Clinical features of common paediatric hip conditions**

	Perthes' disease	DDH	Septic arthritis	Irritable hip	SUFE
Age	4–10 years	From birth	Any age	2–11 years	Teens
Sex	M > F X4	F > M X 7	M > F	M > F	M > F X4 (Never in girls after menarche)
Pyrexia	Apyrexial	Apyrexial	Pyrexial 38 C +	Apyrexial/ modest pyrexia < 37.5C	Apyrexial
Presentation	Painful limp (Hip or knee pain) + reduced range of movement in hip	Not painful	Acute, systemic illness Painful – won't walk	Limping child +/– pain in groin, thigh, and knee	Painful limp Chronic becomes acute
Blood tests	Normal	Normal	FBC (WCC up) ESR up CRP up	FBC (WCC normal) ESR normal CRP normal/a little raised	Normal
Radiology	Plain XR Others 1) MRI 2) Bone scan	USS up to 6 months XR post 6 months	Plain XR Can be normal USS may show fluid MRI shows fluid	USS may show fluid (sterile) XR – normal	XR AP + frog lateral

References

1. Marks DS, Clegg J, Al-Chalabi AN. Routine ultrasound screening for neonatal hip instability. Can it abolish late-presenting congenital dislocation of the hip? *J Bone Joint Surg Br* 1994; **76(4):** 534–8.

2. Broughton NS. Bone and joint infection. In: *A Textbook of Paediatric Orthopaedics*. London: WB Saunders Ltd, 1997.

3. Margetts BM, Perry CA, Taylor JF, Dangerfield PH. The incidence and distribution of Legg-Calve-Perthes' disease in Liverpool 1982–95. *Arch Dis Child* 2001; **84(4):** 351–4.

4. Eldridge J, Dilley A, Austin H, *et al.* The role of protein C, protein S and resistance to activated protein C in Legg–Perthes' disease. *Paediatrics* 2001; **107(6):** 1329–34.

5. Loder RT. Slipped capital femoral epiphysis. [Review Article American Academy of Orthopaedic Surgeons.] AAOS Instructional Course Lecture 2001; **50:** 555–67.

Chapter Six

CHILDREN'S ORTHOPAEDICS IN GENERAL

Alison Edwards and Steven Cutts

Abnormalities of the feet and toes

Congenital talipes equino varus – 'club foot'

The terms CTEV and 'club' foot are currently used interchangeably, although there is an emerging school of thought that claims the term 'club foot' is distasteful and many parents regard the label as stigmatising. The acronym 'CTEV' reminds us that these children have feet that are in equinus; i.e. they attempt to walk on the tip of their big toe (like a horse). Similarly varus reminds us that the foot is turned inwards and also tends to be curved along its length.

The poet, Byron famously had a club foot that was left untreated and did little to impair his lifestyle. All in all, CTEV occurs in about 1 in 1000 Caucasian live births. It is more common in some ethnic groups, such as Polynesians (6.9 per 1000). It may be primary (idiopathic) or secondary (e.g. neuropathic or muscular causes). Sometimes it occurs as part of a syndrome and milder cases may be 'positional'; i.e. the baby's foot was squeezed awkwardly inside the mother's uterus.

The cause of idiopathic club foot is not fully understood. It is more common in boys and half the cases are bilateral. Club foot is also more common in twins. About 25% of patients appear to have a positive family history, usually on their father's side.

We can probably gain some insight into the aetiology of club foot from twin studies. Where one twin is affected by CTEV, an identical twin has a 32% chance of being affected, whereas a non-identical twin has a 3% risk. This information, combined with the data on different ethnic prevalence, would suggest a polygenetic component to the aetiology. However, given that identical twins are known to be genetic clones, it's surprising that the concordance figure isn't even higher. This may be because the intra-uterine environment also plays a role. It must be remembered that club foot sometimes appears to be a

Figure 6.1
Bilateral club feet

Picture shows a five-day-old baby with bilateral club feet. These were syndromic, although the appearance is much the same in idiopathic club foot.

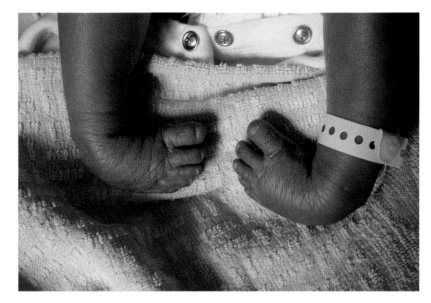

'packaging' problem. For example, club foot is more common in first-born children and following pregnancies that were complicated by oligohydramnios.

With high-resolution ultrasound scanning, many cases are now diagnosed pre-natally and referred via obstetricians. Patients with club foot need referral to a paediatric orthopaedic surgeon. Milder cases are usually managed conservatively with physiotherapy and strapping. Where possible, this process should start within days of birth. The

Figure 6.2
Surgical correction of a club foot

Surgical correction of a club foot (CTEV) through a Cincinnati incision. The medial structures are tight and require lengthening. About 25% of patients will require at least a second operation in later life.

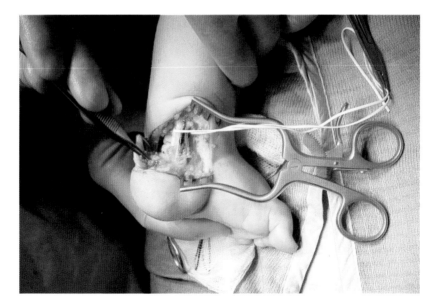

majority, (70–80%) of cases are now managed conservatively. The American surgeon, Ponsetti, has described a technique that uses serial casting and sometimes a minor Achilles tendon operation. These children need to wear splints for up to two years. More severe cases are treated initially with strapping and physiotherapy, with surgery being performed a few months later. The long-term results of surgery are usually satisfactory, although about a quarter of these patients will require at least a second operation later on in childhood or adult life. The occasional, resistant case may even require correction by an Ilizarov frame and a few unfortunate adults with persisting problems require hindfoot fusion.

Biographical note

*During the 1950s, the then unknown Russian doctor, **Gavril Abramovich Ilizarov** (1921–1992) was consulted by a patient with an apparently inoperable deformity in his leg. Assembling an external fixator from a few abandoned bicycle wheels, Ilizarov began a research programme that culminated in the development of an entirely new form of external fixator. To this day, the world centre for Ilizarov research is based in the former Soviet city of Kurgan. Because of the restrictions of the Cold War, his work remained unrecognised in the West for many years until a group of Italian doctors visited Kurgan in 1981 and went on to popularise the technique in the West. Ilizarov frames are most famously used for leg lengthening operations (for example in patients of limited stature), although they are also used to correct particularly difficult deformities (such as resistant club foot).*

With modern treatment, almost all patients with CTEV can ultimately lead a near normal life, running around with friends and playing sports at school. It is, however, worth emphasising to the parents that the foot will probably never look entirely normal and the child will be unable to become a performance athlete. One of the more annoying problems is the varus angulation of the toes, which never seems to go away. In addition, there is often a longer-term difference in the shape of the calves, with the affected side appearing wasted in relation to the normal side. The club foot itself may always remain smaller than the normal side and sometimes even the tibia is shorter on the affected

Figure 6.3
Ilizarov frame for the correction of a club foot

In the case of a patient at puberty with a club foot that has resisted full correction during earlier interventions, an Ilizarov frame may represent the final treatment option. The bolts are turned through 360 degrees, advancing the rods by 1mm daily. Over a period of two months, the deformity may be sufficiently corrected.

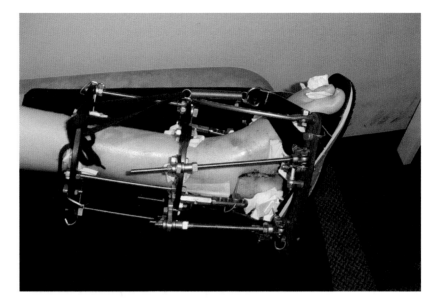

Figure 6.4
'Successfully' corrected club foot

Note that the affected foot is smaller than the normal foot. The calf is hypoplastic and the tibia slightly shorter compared to the normal leg. The toes are swept in a varus direction. These changes will remain with the patient for life.

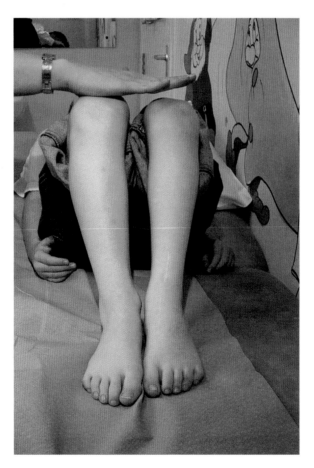

side. This odd collection of changes remind us that CTEV seems to be having an impact on the development of the limb as a whole and is clearly much more than a simple packaging defect.

Hallux valgus in childhood and adolescence

In hallux valgus the big toe has swung laterally and the head of the big toe metatarsal is unusually prominent. In many cases the forefoot has actually widened; i.e. the patient has a 'splayed' forefoot. We tend to associate this condition with much older adults, but it can occur in children and teenagers. Girls, in particular, may find wearing fashionable footwear difficult. It's often claimed that in countries where people cannot afford shoes, hallux valgus doesn't exist. Interesting though this anecdote may be, the option of going barefoot is unrealistic in the modern world.

Adolescent hallux valgus often has a strong family history and many teenage patients may be accompanied by anxious relatives who suffered from the same problem. Hallux valgus is more common in girls than boys due, in part, to the shape of ladies' shoes. The teenagers themselves are more likely to complain of the cosmetic deformity than the pain. Remember that even quite severe looking hallux valgus may not be associated with any pain.

In an older adult, we can try to blame a problem like hallux valgus on the toil of the passing years. We have to look for other explanations in a child. On examination you may discover that young patients suffer from generalised ligamentous laxity. Symptoms are unusual in a child or teenager and some surgeons believe than bunion surgery in children and adolescents should be delayed until the growth plates have fused. Even when surgery is attempted, the results may be disappointing. The deformity may recur in later life and may even become painful because of the surgery.

A medial arch support may help provide some correction. Osteotomy is best delayed as long as possible. Pain or ulceration under the toes would be regarded as more convincing indications for surgery than cosmesis.

Overriding toes

Congenital elevation of the little toe with rotation causes the little toe to sit on top of the fourth toe, sometimes resulting in painful corns on the sole of the feet. Strapping may correct this and surgery can realign the soft tissues if symptoms are a problem.

Curly toes

In this condition, the fourth and fifth toes are flexed and medially rotated at the distal interphalangeal joint. This is also discussed on page 101.

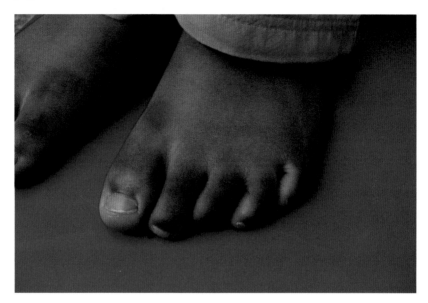

Figure 6.5
Curly toes

This child has curly toes. Although they may be tolerated by the patient and their parents, they can be easily corrected by a flexor tenotomy, which can be performed as a day case under general anaesthetic.

Back pain in children

In adults, low back pain is usually self-limiting and as a rule does not demand investigation. In children it is more of a concern. Less than 2% per cent of paediatric referrals are for back pain. It's unusual for a child to invent the symptoms of back pain and symptoms **must** be taken seriously. It is more common in boys than girls and reaches a peak at ages 13 to 15.

In children under four, always consider infection or tumour as possible causes, and check the ESR, FBC, and CRP. It is worth noting that lymphocytic leukaemia actually presents with back pain in 6% of cases.

Adolescents with back pain are more likely to have spondylolysis or Scheuermann's kyphosis. Pain from Scheuermann's kyphosis is localised to the mid line in the scapula area, and presents in teenagers (usually boys) with poor posture rather than pain. Painful scoliosis may signify a tumour or spinal cord anomaly and should be referred.

Biographical note

In 1920, **HW Scheuermann** *(1877–1960), a Danish orthopaedic surgeon, submitted a PhD thesis about a 'new' form of juvenile thoracic kyphosis to the University of Copenhagen. It was rejected. In spite of this, the condition still bears his name, although one should add that it had been previously described by Schanz in 1911.*

Spina bifida

Spina bifida is a congenital problem with the spine in which some of the posterior structures are missing. Some patients are born with an obvious defect on the base of the spine and there may even be exposed nervous tissue. Clearly, these patients will suffer from lifelong neurological problems. However, spina bifida occulta is a much milder form of the condition. It is surprisingly common and may even be asymptomatic; indeed, it is easily undiagnosed. It is often associated with a hairy patch on the skin in the small of the back. In these cases, the spinal cord and meninges are almost normal, but there is an underlying vertebral defect that may only be picked up incidentally on spinal X-rays.

Spina bifida may also be associated with many foot deformities. When a child presents with a foot deformity it is essential to examine the small of the back. A small hairy patch may point to the underlying problem. About 2.5 per 1000 live births are affected and there are unexplained geographical variations. Antenatal screening for spina bifida is now possible by measuring alpha fetoprotein. For this reason, the number of live births suffering from severe spina bifida has decreased substantially in modern times.

Osteochondritic conditions

Several bones in the body are affected by osteochondritis. In osteochondritis, there is damage, fragmentation, or separation of articular cartilage and bone. Sometimes the condition seems to be multifocal and can run in families. These conditions usually present during a period of rapid growth and are most common during the early teens.

There are three broad categories of osteochondritis:

1. Crushing e.g. Frieberg's (forefoot), Panner disease (elbow).
2. Splitting e.g. Osteochondritis dissecans of the knee.
3. Pulling e.g. Osgood-Schlatter (knee) and Sever's (heel).

We will consider the third type, i.e. 'pulling' (or 'traction' forms) of osteochondritis here.

One of the key differences between the adult skeleton and the paediatric skeleton is the presence of 'growth plates' in children. Growth plates are usually weaker than in the fully ossified adult and this can cause problems where strong tendons insert very close to a growth plate. The calf muscles insert through the Achilles tendon into the back of the calcaneum very close to a growth plate. Although the muscles of teenage children approach adult strength, the skeleton is not yet fully mature.

This creates a problem in **Sever's disease**, which represents a form of traction osteochondritis. In Sever's disease, the Achilles tendon appears to be trying to pull the heel growth plate open. A tender swelling forms on the back of the heel.

Similarly, in **Osgood–Schlatter disease,** the quadriceps muscle tries to 'pull off' the tibial tubercle from the underlying growth plate. The quadriceps muscle effectively inserts into the tibial tubercle via the patella ligament. Once the pubertal growth spurt ends, the growth plates close over and the problem usually goes away. For this reason, Osgood–Schlatter disease is a *self-limiting* condition typically affecting physically active youngsters over the age of ten. It is caused by recurrent micro-trauma to the area of bone where the patella tendon inserts.

Patients complain of pain and swelling over the tibial tubercle, often bilaterally. As in Sever's disease, symptoms are exacerbated by activity and resolve with rest. Surgery is not advised unless a painful bony swelling still persists just below the knee after growth ceases. Parents should be reassured that the condition will settle on its own over about a year, and the child should avoid painful activities. Management is with simple painkillers. Many teenagers simply continue to play through the pain. Immobilisation with a plaster cylinder can be tried in severe cases but is usually tolerated poorly. Surgical attempts to remove a swelling that persists into adult life are often requested in girls, although the results of such adventures are often disappointing.

Popliteal cysts

The popliteal cyst in a child usually presents as a soft fluctuant swelling in the popliteal fossa, most evident with the knee in extension. Unlike a Baker's cyst, there is no associated intra-articular pathology. The cyst is actually a semi-membranous bursa. Surgery is rarely performed as there is a very high recurrence rate after aspiration and most resolve spontaneously.

Dislocating/subluxing patella[3]

Some teenagers suffer from recurrent patella subluxation. It often affects tall teenage girls. They may describe a patella that dislocated and then spontaneously relocated after a fall. Sometimes they had to attend A&E to have it reduced under sedation. After a dislocation, the knee may be very swollen for a few weeks afterwards. Once the acute swelling and pain has subsided they can be reassessed.

The patella almost always dislocates laterally. In fact, the patella spends its entire life trying to dislocate laterally. This is because it is trapped within the tendon on the quadriceps muscle, which has an oblique pull upwards *and* outwards from the knee. Nature has tried to avoid dislocation by having a prominent lateral femoral condyle that mechanically blocks dislocation. However, on skyline view X-rays some of these patients often have too shallow a grove in the femur, which makes dislocation easier. They may also have general ligamentous laxity or an abnormal Q angle, i.e. the quadriceps pull is particularly oblique.

To begin with, we would try to treat these patients with physiotherapy to strengthen the *vastus medialis* muscle (VMO exercises), to try to oppose the lateral pull of the rest of the quadriceps. Strapping may also help. In the case of recurrent dislocation, various operations have been developed, all of which inflict scars on girls of a sensitive age. Nowadays, we can do some of these arthroscopically, e.g. by lateral release. Unfortunately, this kind of adolescent problem predisposes to PFJ pain in later life.

Normal variants in paediatric orthopaedics

Children often develop minor orthopaedic abnormalities, which are part of the normal spectrum of development. Such problems are often a source of great parental concern, although most are self-correcting. The children themselves remain unconcerned about minor problems such as slight in-toeing, which often self-corrects with time, and the real anxiety lies in the minds of the parents!

Minor abnormalities as described here probably don't require automatic referral, although many parents prefer the reassurance of a hospital specialist. The medical anxiety is that the problem may reflect a more profound underlying condition. In practice the decision to refer a child for specialist opinion lies with the individual doctor in the primary-care setting. However, certain themes are worth remembering. For example, pes cavus (high arched foot) is far more likely to need investigating than pes planus (flat feet), which is almost always benign. Abnormalities that appear to be associated with other problems, such as short stature, are more alarming and are more likely to justify a specialist referral. Similarly, significant delays in reaching major milestones are a cause for greater concern.

Box 6.1   **Normal walking ages and developmental milestones**

9 months	sits without support
12 months	walks with one hand support
15 months	walks alone
2 years	climbs stairs and runs
4 years	stands on one leg
5 years	hops

It is normal to be walking alone by the age of 14 months, but there is no need to be concerned up to the age of 18 months.

In-toeing[5]

In-toeing is one of the commonest reasons for referral to a paediatric orthopaedic clinic. It should be remembered that the rotational profile of a child's legs is not fixed until about the age of seven.

If a child is in-toeing, the lower limb must be rotated somewhere along its length. There are three reasons why a child may be in-toeing and these tend to be age-specific (Table 6.1).

Table 6.1   **Common causes of in-toeing**

Rotation	Condition	Age
A twist in the forefoot	Metatarsus adductus	First few months of life
Tibia	Internal tibial torsion	Toddlers (1–3 years old)
Femur	Femoral anteversion	3–10 years old

Metatarsus adductus
In metatarsus adductus the medial border of the forefoot is curved

inwards. This is thought to be due to over-activity in the abductor hallucis muscle and may be noticed in the first few months of life.

Treatment for metatarsus adductus is to advise against prone nursing – watch and wait. The vast majority spontaneously resolve if they are flexible and can be passively corrected. Persistence beyond the age of five years or rigid deformity may require surgery. Metatarsus adductus tends to be associated with other problems such as DDH. Therefore, the hips must always be re-examined in a case of metatarsus adductus.

Internal tibial torsion

The patient presenting with internal tibial torsion is usually a toddler. As with metatarsus adductus, most cases spontaneously resolve. Attempts at accelerating resolution with various unsightly splints are probably not worthwhile. In a tiny proportion of children a derotational osteotomy may be required. This would usually be delayed until at least 8–10 years of age to give maximum time for natural correction.

Internal femoral torsion

In an adult the typical angle of anteversion of the femoral neck is 15 degrees. However, a baby is born with an angle of 40 degrees. For this reason, in most children there must be a gradual transition of the angle towards the adult value. In some children the angle persists into early childhood and these present aged three to ten years with an unseemly gait and symmetrical in-toeing.

A child with an increased angle of anteversion of the femoral neck will have a reduced or absent external rotation to the hip. Complete absence of external rotation is a particularly bad prognostic sign while 15 degrees of external rotation is considered adequate. Once again the natural history is one of spontaneous resolution. A small minority require rotational osteotomy in their teens. Another group self-compensate by developing external rotation of the tibia so that the feet point forward normally with the patella pointing inwards – the so called **squinting patella syndrome**. This is cosmetically unattractive. However, it would require bilateral femoral *and* tibial osteotomies to correct and is probably best ignored.

Bow legs

A baby is born with bow legs when the knee joint is in varus. However, during the course of the child's normal growth and development the knee gradually straightens and by the age of three to eight years the knee will have returned to a valgus angle. The adult angle is said to be seven degrees of valgus.

The bowing of early childhood is **symmetrical** and improves steadily. Splintage makes no difference to the progress of the condition.

Pathological bowing may be **asymmetrical**, it deteriorates with time, and tends to be more severe than physiological bowing.

Causes of pathological bowing
- Blount's disease
- rickets
- skeletal dysplasias
- trauma

> Biographical note
>
> **Walter Putnam Blount** *(1900–1992), American orthopaedic surgeon. Grandson of the American Civil War surgeon, Joseph Blount. Chief orthopaedic surgeon at Milwaukee's Children's Hospital. In 1957, as Professor of Orthopaedics at Marquette Medical School, Blount described a special form of tibia vara seen in African-American children.*

Blount's disease is a form of tibia vara that usually affects children of African–Caribbean descent, although it can also affect Caucasian children, and is associated with childhood obesity. Blount's disease is bilateral in 60% of cases. The growth plate just below the knee seems to stop growing on the medial side whilst the lateral side continues to grow. This produces a bow leg. Bowing with short stature suggests skeletal dysplasia.

When requesting X-rays for the lower limb remember to state that they are to be taken AP and lateral and weight bearing.

Knock knees – genu valgum

In knock knees the legs are in valgus. Beyond the age of about three years, valgus knees are normal, but an increased or asymmetric angle may be pathological. Whilst most cases tend to resolve with growth, severe and asymmetric cases may not. A previous fracture affecting the growth plate may lead to genu valgum, as can skeletal dysplasias and rickets developed later in childhood.

Surgery can be performed in severe cases and is usually aimed at causing partial and usually temporary arrest of the growth plate in order to create a compensatory asymmetric growth to bring the limb back into alignment. This procedure is often unpopular with patients and their families, as it may take some time for the correction to occur. A residual angle at the end of the pubertal growth spurt would require an osteotomy.

Flat feet

The child presenting with a foot problem is likely to be there at the request of the parents. It's useful to have a clear understanding of how normal feet behave. When the normal standing child is examined from behind, the heels should be in slight valgus. However, when the child stands on tip-toe, the heels go into varus and the longitudinal arch of the foot becomes exaggerated.

Flat feet are normal in young children. The arches develop gradually with growth and do not normally appear until about six years of age. Children who have generalised ligamentous laxity are more likely to have delayed arches. Some doctors argue that flat feet may be physiological up to the age of ten years.

Studies on both military recruits and 'normal' civilian populations[4] suggest that flexible flat feet do not increase the risk of foot pain compared with those with normal arches. Of course, flat feet may be pathological.

Pathological causes of flat feet
- hypermobility syndromes
- cerebral palsy (CP)
- tarsal coalitions

The tip-toe test. If the child stands on tip-toe, the long flexor tendons become tense and the arches appear.

Jack's test. Similarly, lifting the big toe off the ground produces the arch in a mobile foot and this can be very reassuring for parents and the doctor.

Treatment
Although there is often significant parental pressure to provide some form of active treatment, reassurance is usually all that is needed in

patients with flexible flat feet. Arch supports may improve the lifespan of the child's shoes.[6] An arch support will not, of course, change the natural history of the condition. Where the deformity is rigid, or painful, then further investigation may be warranted.

Tarsal coalitions

Here, two or three of the small tarsal bones in the hindfoot have failed to fully separate. There may be a bony or cartilaginous bar between the calcaneus and navicular or talus and calcaneus.

This problem usually presents at age 10 to 11 years. Coalitions are a common cause of painful flat feet and the pain is worse after activity. The subtalar joint is not mobile. There is often a family history of the problem and the incidence has been estimated at 1% of the population, although a proportion of these people are completely asymptomatic. The more painful cases require surgery to release the connecting bar of tissue.

Paralytic flat feet

Associated with several neurological conditions, including CP and spina bifida.

Pes cavus – high arch foot

Pes cavus is not a disease, it's a physical sign. Unlike flat feet, pes cavus must be considered pathological until proven otherwise.

In pes cavus, the longitudinal arch of the foot is elevated and there is often associated clawing of the toes. The metatarsal heads are more prominent than normal and in persistent pes cavus there may be callosities over the metatarsal heads. The priority is to determine the underlying cause of the condition and then determine the best treatment/prognosis. Some cases are idiopathic, but others reflect real pathology.

Always perform a thorough neurological examination in pes cavus.

Always inspect the base of the spine for a hairy patch (spina bifida occulta) in pes cavus.

There are two types of high arched feet:
1. pure cavus
2. cavovarus feet.

In pure cavus feet there is no varus or valgus deformity to the hindfoot. In a cavovarus foot the deformity is associated with a varus hindfoot. For example, idiopathic pes cavus is usually a pure pes cavus, whereas neurological pes cavus is usually cavovarus.

Causes of pes cavus

Pes cavus is a physical sign, not a disease. It has many causes:

- idiopathic
- neuromuscular, e.g. Duchenne muscular dystrophy, Charcot–Marie–Tooth disease or CP
- central neurological problem, e.g. Friedrich's ataxia
- it may reflect a spinal cord abnormality
- polio.

The age of the patient gives a clue to the aetiology.

Adolescent pes cavus is usually idiopathic. There is often a family history. It is associated with claw toes, tender callosities, pain at the metatarsal heads. Occasionally, mild hereditary motor and sensory neuropathies are missed until adolescence.

Childhood pes cavus is usually neuromuscular. Sometimes the shoes have worn out awkwardly. There may be callosities over the metatarsal heads and if the pathology is neuropathic there may be painless ulcers on the heads of the metatarsals.

Toe walking

For many children, toe walking is a normal part of their development.

Figure 6.6
**Idiopathic
toe walking**

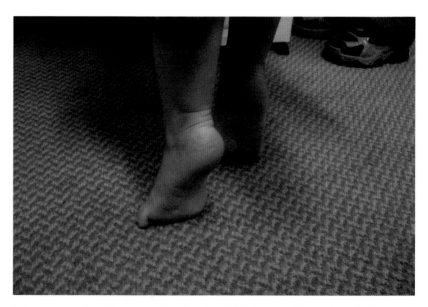

This three-year-old child occasionally walks with a flat foot but mostly remains on her toes. There is no neurology; the problem is symmetrical and bilateral and was not preceded by a period of normal walking, i.e. it began when the infant started walking. This condition will almost certainly resolve without active treatment.

Physiological toe walking is usually intermittent and may be followed by a period of flat foot strike before the child switches to a normal heel strike.

Very occasionally, in persistent cases, surgical lengthening of the Achilles tendon may be effective. However, persistent toe walking may self-correct up to the age of ten and, for this reason, many orthopaedic surgeons choose to delay surgery as long as possible.

Children who initially walk normally and subsequently develop toe walking are demonstrating **pathological toe walking** and this requires urgent referral. There are several causes of this, some of which may cause the child to toe walk from the beginning.

Causes of pathological toe walking

- diplegic CP
- Duchenne muscular dystrophy
- hereditary and sensory motor neuropathy
- spinal dysraphism

Spinal dysraphism is a developmental abnormality in the spine affecting the spinal cord. Unilateral toe walking is almost always pathological.

Causes of unilateral toe walking

- hemiplegic CP
- DDH

In a child with abnormal feet and gait it is mandatory to examine the base of the spine. A hairy patch may reveal previously undiagnosed spina bifida occulta.

Duchenne muscular dystrophy (or the milder form, Becker muscular dystrophy) is an important diagnosis to exclude (key test = plasma CPK). It is sex-linked (i.e. it is found on the Y chromosome) and therefore only found in boys. Although Duchenne is impossible to cure, the parents of the child may be planning more children and any delay in diagnosis may affect genetic counselling.

Curly toes

Curly toes are often bilateral. The fourth and fifth toes are the most commonly involved. They are usually asymptomatic but can run in families. Parents may be concerned about children developing the same problems that they had. Severe/painful cases may benefit from surgical correction, usually in the form of a simple flexor tenotomy.

Growing pains and night cramps[7]

Fifteen per cent of children wake up at night complaining of night pain. The pain is usually only present at night and has resolved in the morning. In daylight the child does not limp. There is no neurology. The family may have noticed that the symptoms are relieved by massage and simple analgesics. Most cases are regarded as idiopathic and require no treatment.

There are also sinister causes of nocturnal leg pain, including some tumours. For example, osteoid osteoma is a classic example of a benign tumour which causes more pain at night than in the day. Night pain in association with a discernable soft tissue or bony lump is alarming and should be referred urgently.

Differential diagnoses for rare causes of night pain

Osteoid osteoma is a simple benign tumour of bone, it is characteristically more painful at night. The pain, however, would be unilateral.

Leukaemia may be associated with bilateral leg pain. The diagnosis can often be made by a FBC.

References

1. Macnicol MF. The management of club foot: issues for debate. *J Bone Joint Surgery Am* 2003; **85**: 167–70.
2. Broughton NS. *Spina Bifida: a textbook of paediatric orthopaedics*. London: Saunders Publications, 1997; Chapter 9.
3. Broughton NS. *Spina Bifida: a textbook of paediatric orthopaedics*. London: Saunders Publications, 1997; Chapter 19.
4. Hogan MT, Staheli LT. Arch height and lower limb pain: an adult civilian study. *Foot and Ankle Int* 2002; **23(1)**: 43–7.
5. Kling TF, Hensinger RN. Angular and torsional deformities of the limbs of children. *Clinical Orthop* 1983; **186**: 136–42.
6. Wenger D, Maudlin D, Speck G, *et al*. Corrective shoes and inserts as treatment for flexible flat feet in infants and children. *J Bone Joint Surgery Am* 1989; **71A**: 800–10.
7. Baxter A, Dulberg C. Growing pains in children. *J Paediatric Orthopaedics* 1988; **8**: 402–6.

Chapter Seven

THE PAEDIATRIC SPINE

Steven Cutts, Darren Clarke, and Alison Edwards

Key points

- Most causes of scoliosis are quite benign.
- Childhood curvatures will usually stop progressing at the end of puberty.
- Only the most severe curvatures of the spine threaten cardiovascular or respiratory function.
- Surgery for scoliosis is not without risk and requires a specialist spinal surgeon.
- Consider systemic conditions that may be associated with spinal deformity.

The paediatric spine and scoliosis

Scoliosis refers to a lateral curvature in the spine. *Scoliosis is a physical sign* – it is not a disease. There are many causes of scoliosis and fortunately most of these are quite benign.

Kyphosis refers to a spinal curvature in the antero–posterior plane. Some diseases present with a pure kyphotic curve (e.g. Scheuermann's). However, many children have a three-dimensional deformity and are therefore said to have **kyphoscoliosis.**

Spinal deformity in children is not a condition that must be reported, so accurate figures for prevalence are not available. It is known that about 1 in 500 children suffer from progressive adolescent idiopathic scoliosis and some of these may require surgery.

Examination of the scoliotic child

Spinal curvature is often part of a broader clinical picture, so it's important to look for signs of other medical conditions. For example, scoliosis with short stature suggests skeletal dysplasia. Multiple 'café-au-lait' spots may indicate neurofibromatosis. In any child with a spinal problem, it is mandatory to examine the base of the spine. A patch of hair or a skin dimple in the lumbar region may indicate spina bifida (see Chapter 6). The curve itself may be confined to the lumbar or

Table 7.1   **Comparison of infantile and adolescent scoliosis**

Type	Sex	Region	Direction	Outcome
Infantile scoliosis	60% male Male > female	Thoracic/ lumbar	Convex to the left	Spontaneous resolution possible
Adolescent scoliosis	90% female Female > male	Usually thoracic	Convex to the right	No resolution/ deteriorates

thoracic region but may extend across the thoraco-lumbar spine. It's also worth checking for a difference in leg length and for deformities in the foot and ankle.

Figure 7.1
Spina bifida

A small hairy patch of skin at the base of the spine is the tell-tale sign of spina bifida occulta. This young male has bilateral clawing of the toes and high-arched feet. He is ambulant with the help of crutches and callipers.

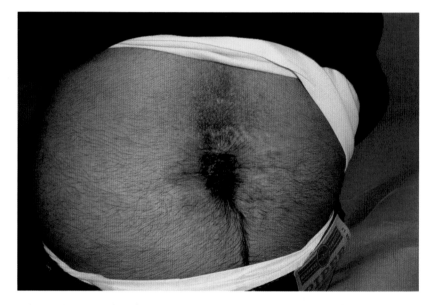

Non-structural and structural scoliosis

In some patients, the structure of the spine is normal, but the child develops a curve secondary to a problem elsewhere. The simplest example of this would be asymmetric leg lengths or a pelvic tilt. These patients are sometimes described as having a **postural** or **non-structural scoliosis**. When the child sits down, the scoliosis vanishes. In other patients, the problem is intrinsic to the spine and cannot be corrected by any manoeuvre by the examiner. This is a **structural scoliosis** and often exists in three dimensions.

Adolescent idiopathic scoliosis

Adolescent idiopathic scoliosis is a three-dimensional, structural scoliosis. It is by far the most common form of scoliosis and when we speak of 'scoliosis', we are usually speaking of adolescent idiopathic scoliosis. It can be detected or emphasised by Adam's test. Here, the patient is asked to bend forwards and the examiner looks for a telltale rib hump. The hump represents an asymmetry in the rib cage caused by the rotation of the vertebra. As the initial curve progresses, the child may develop two adjacent secondary curves producing an S-shaped spine. Adolescent idiopathic scoliosis often progresses rapidly during the pubertal growth spurt. It is not normally painful.

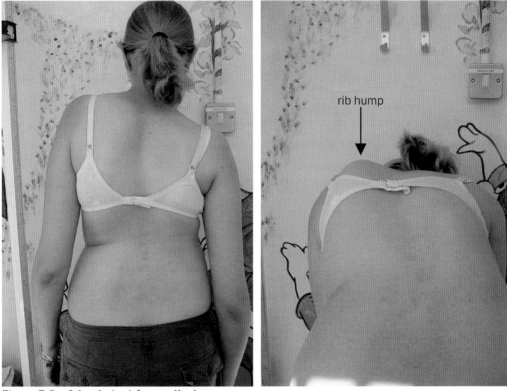

rib hump

Figure 7.2   Adam's test for scoliosis
(a)   (b)
It is easiest to spot scoliosis with the patient standing with their back to you. This girl's scoliotic curve is visible in the upright position (a), but it becomes more obvious when she leans forward (b). This is an example of three-dimensional scoliosis with rotation of the spine and consequent rib hump.

Luckily, most childhood and teenage curvatures of the spine will stop progressing at the end of the pubertal growth spurt. If we're confident that the pubertal growth spurt is about to end and the curve is minor, we can probably leave it untreated. However, if the child is much younger with many years of growth ahead of them, there is more cause for concern. In the assessment of a child with a three-dimensional scoliotic deformity it is therefore important to consider a fourth dimension – time.

An influential study performed in Iowa[1] suggested that a thoracic curve of 30 degrees or less will not progress once the growth spurt has ended.

Key points

- Scoliosis is a physical sign, not a disease.
- Accurate figures for prevalence are not available.
- Non-structural and structural scoliosis can easily be distinguished.
- Idiopathic scoliosis can be detected or emphasised by Adam's test.

Adolescent idiopathic scoliosis affects girls eight times more frequently than boys and typically produces a right-sided thoracic curve. It is best to screen for adolescent idiopathic scoliosis when the child is about ten years old. About 4% of the teenage population are affected. One problem in defining such figures is that few of us will have an entirely straight spine and, as always in orthopaedics, a threshold level has to be chosen for defining the condition. A degree of curvature of at least seven degrees or more is sometimes quoted as a significant deformity.

What causes idiopathic scoliosis?

In the past, 'idiopathic scoliosis' was used as a blanket term for all unexplained spinal curves. Thanks to MRI scanning, quite a few 'idiopathic' patients now turn out to have obvious spinal pathology. The remaining, 'true' idiopathic scoliotics offer other clues to their aetiology. For example, idiopathic scoliotics are taller than their peers. In addition, their overall skeletal maturity is retarded by about 12 to 18 months. This suggests a multi-factorial inheritance affecting the whole skeleton.

Some specialists believe that idiopathic scoliosis represents altered body symmetry; for example, teenage girls with scoliosis sometimes have asymmetric breasts and occasionally require corrective plastic surgery.

Key points

- In assessment of scoliosis it is important to consider the dimension of time.
- About 4% of the teenage population have adolescent idiopathic scoliosis.
- It is now often possible to identify a cause for what was previously thought to be idiopathic scoliosis.

Progression and danger signs

Adolescent idiopathic scoliosis either remains the same or deteriorates as the child grows. It will not spontaneously resolve. At skeletal maturity the curve will stop progressing. Most patients are simply kept under regular observation. In a small minority, the condition will be so severe as to require surgery.

Scoliosis that begins in a younger child is more worrying because there is more time available for progression. Most thoracic curves in idiopathic scoliosis are typically convex to the right. A high proportion of thoracic curves that are convex to the left are likely to reflect definitive neurogenic pathology. Similarly, spinal curvature is more of a concern in a boy than a girl. This is because, statistically, spinal curvature in a boy is more likely to be associated with threatening pathology. These patients therefore deserve to be investigated by MRI scanning. Sadly, very severe curves, that is those over 50 degrees, may continue to progress at about one degree per year during adult life.

Patient concerns

Even minor scoliotic curves can be distressing for the teenage patient. Some of the more severe ones can be quite alarming and it is tempting to suggest that severe scoliosis ought to lead to cardiovascular and respiratory compromise. Luckily, such crippling complications are rare. Unfortunately, a child afflicted by scoliosis before the age of eight is at considerable risk of impaired pulmonary development and these children are also believed to be at risk of premature death in adult life.[2] A curve of over 30 degrees can be shown to cause significant ventilation and perfusion (VQ) abnormalities in the adult. These patients often require formal lung function tests before corrective surgery.

Many teenage girls and their parents are concerned that they will not be able to have children because they have scoliosis. Broadly speaking, this is not the case. Because idiopathic scoliosis has a multifactorial aetiology, the risk of any children being affected by the condition is small.

Key points

- Idiopathic scoliosis may either remain stable or deteriorate as the child grows.
- Most thoracic curves in idiopathic scoliosis are typically convex to the right. Curves to the left need investigating.
- The fear that girls with scoliosis will not be able to have children is largely unfounded.
- Danger signs include severe curves in the young, scoliosis in boys, thoracic curves convex to the left, and scoliosis that is painful or associated with neurological signs.

Radiographic investigations and treatment

Children with scoliosis are often X-rayed repeatedly. To try to avoid this repeated radiation exposure, a technique of photographing the torso under special horizontal strips of light has been developed. However, this method of assessment has never surpassed plain X-rays, and in some of the centres where it was tried it has already been abandoned.

MRI scanning has transformed our understanding of scoliosis and as this investigation becomes more readily available, it is likely that all scoliotic children will receive an MRI scan in the future.

Bracing

It is unlikely that bracing has ever cured a scoliotic child, although some experts believe that bracing can stop a curve progressing. Unfortunately, many teenagers only wear their braces when attending outpatient clinics. Such poor compliance may explain the poor results of bracing. Modern orthotists have managed to produce lightweight braces that are less stigmatising for children to wear and it is hoped that this will lead to an improvement in compliance. Remember that, if nothing else, bracing represents a well-intended attempt to evade the risks of surgery.

Surgery in scoliosis

When a child with a curved spine presents in primary care, it is reasonable to refer those with significant scoliosis to a regional orthopaedic surgeon. To a certain extent this is a subjective judgement on the part of the referring doctor. However, curves of more than seven degrees are regarded as significant by spinal surgeons. In addition, curves that

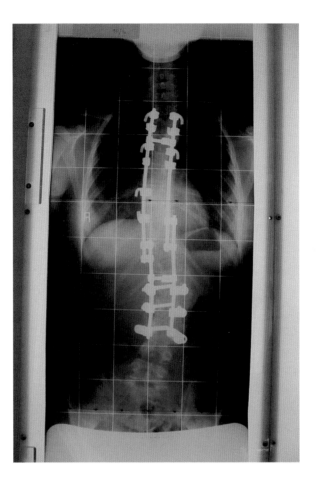

are convex to the left, curves found in boys, and curves found in chil-dren or younger teenagers should raise alarm bells. Most of these refer-rals will result in reassurance for the patient and relatives.

In any case, non-structural scoliosis does not require spinal surgery, although it might benefit from the skills of a paediatric orthopaedic surgeon.

The risks of surgery

Surgery in scoliosis is expensive and carries some risks, including the risk of catastrophic paralysis. For this reason, corrective surgery is reserved for carefully selected patients. It would not be appropriate to offer surgery for a trivial curve appearing at the end of adolescence. After instrumentation and fusion, the spine will have a reduced range of movement. In any event, the rib hump, which is often the patient's main concern, will probably persist.

Figure 7.4
Scoliosis braces

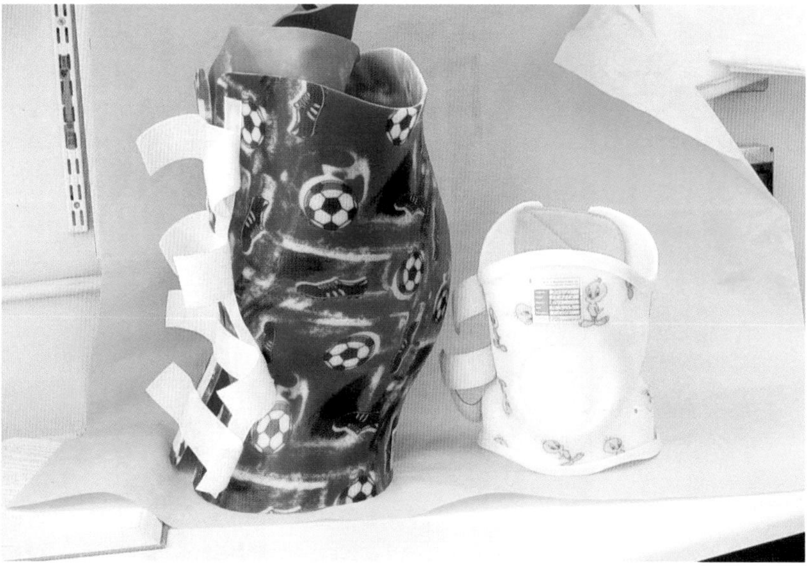

During the adolescent growth spurt, scoliosis can be treated by bracing. It's unlikely that bracing can cure scoliosis but it can probably stop progression of the curve. Bracing is critically dependent on patient compliance, which may not be high amongst teenagers, although the advent of lightweight, colourful and patterned bracing materials will help in this regard.

Who should operate?

Spinal surgery to correct scoliosis requires the skills of a specialist consultant, and the number of these is limited. In October 2001, there were 30 spinal surgeons in the UK and Republic of Ireland undertaking the management of spinal deformity.[3] Some centres have actually given up performing scoliosis correction because they can no longer obtain the financial and/or human resources. Some consultants only perform ten operative procedures per year, whilst others perform over a hundred.

Key points

- Photographic assessment of scoliosis progression has largely been abandoned in favour of plain X-rays.
- Early-onset scoliosis should be scanned by MRI.
- Most orthopaedic referrals will simply result in reassurance for the patient and their families.
- Surgical correction of scoliosis carries a small risk of neurological injury, including paraplegia.

Infantile and adolescent scolioses

Infantile and adolescent scolioses have a number of different character-istics. Infantile idiopathic scoliosis affects babies in the first three months of life. There is a recognised association with plagiocephaly (flattening of the back or side of the head). The pattern of the infantile disease is the reverse of adolescent scoliosis with the typical curve being convex to the left and boys outnumbering girls. A rotatory de-formity produces a rib hump. Infantile scoliosis usually resolves within three years and rarely requires treatment.

Scheuermann's kyphosis

This form of kyphosis was first described by Scheuermann in 1920 and is a painless condition typically affecting teenage boys. A previously well child becomes round shouldered and the patient develops a fixed kyphotic deformity in the thoracic spine that cannot be corrected. It is more obvious when viewed in profile with the patient leaning forward. When you examine the backs of the thighs, the hamstrings are often tight. Like many developmental deformities of the spine, most cases do not require treatment. The kyphosis usually stops progressing at the end of the pubertal growth spurt. Severe cases are sometimes treated with bracing before the skeleton matures. The worst cases may develop pain or even neurological problems. Surgery is usually regarded as in-appropriate for what is typically a cosmetic deformity, but is occasion-ally performed.

Systemic conditions associated with spinal deformity

Scoliosis may be associated with other pathologies and there are well-recognised warning signs that may indicate them. A child complaining of back pain that is worse at night may have an osteoid osteoma. Neu-rofibromatosis is associated with scoliosis and may present in the child with 'café-au-lait' spots. About 50% of children with Marfan's syn-drome get scoliosis. Osteogenesis imperfecta is also associated with sco-liosis and is usually managed conservatively. Surgical correction in this particular group of patients is technically difficult because instruments cannot grip on the soft bone.

Spina bifida is also often associated with spinal deformity, often in conjunction with altered neurology. Scoliosis is a well-known feature of quadriplegic CP. Children with CP usually come with a plethora of other medical problems, although corrective surgery is still sometimes performed.

Figure 7.5
Spina bifida feet

The picture shows the condition affecting the patient's left side more prominently. There is a tightness of the Achilles tendon, a partially sensate foot and clawing in the toes.

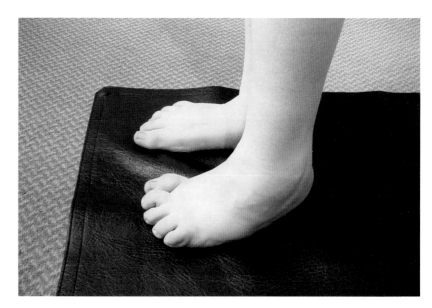

Duchenne muscular dystrophy

Duchenne is one of the most sinister conditions to be associated with spinal deformity. Whilst impossible to cure, it is important to reach an early diagnosis to allow genetic counselling of the parents. However, by the time spinal deformity appears the children are usually over the age of 11 and already wheelchair bound. Surgery is occasionally performed to maintain a straight spine and to delay respiratory failure in the final years of life.

Back pain in children

Back pain in adults is common and rarely serious. Back pain in children is unusual and should always be taken seriously. Prepubertal children rarely 'invent' back pain, and if a child complains of back pain for more than two weeks then they should be investigated.[4] Baseline studies would include FBC, ESR, and CRP. If inflammatory pathology is suspected, then a rheumatoid screen, anti-nuclear antibodies, and HLA B27 testing may be useful. In children, back pain may be associated with spinal infection (including TB) and malignancy.

Key points

- 20–40% of patients with neurofibromatosis develop spinal deformity.
- Duchenne muscular dystrophy is one of the most sinister associations of spinal deformity.
- Persistent back pain in children should always be taken seriously.
- Scheuermann's kyphosis is a painless condition that typically affects teenage boys and most cases need no treatment.

References

1. Weinstein SL, Zavala DC, Ponseti IV. Idiopathic scoliosis. Long-term follow-up and prognosis in untreated patients. *J Bone Joint Surg Am* 1981; **63A**: 702–12.

2. Siegler D, Zorab PA. The influence of lung volume on gas transfer in scoliosis. *Br J Dis Chest* 1982; **76(1)**: 44–50.

3. The management of spinal deformity in the United Kingdom, Guide to Practice can be found at www.boa.ac.uk/PDF%20files/Management%20of%20spinal%20deformity%20in%20UK.pdf

4. Thompson GH. Back pain in children. [Review] Chapter 22 American Academy of Orthopaedic Surgeons Instructional Course Lecture. 1994; **43**: 221–30.

Chapter Eight

CEREBRAL PALSY

Steven Cutts, Graham Myers, and Alison Edwards

Key points

- Antenatal and obstetric care have improved, but the incidence of CP remains unchanged.
- The initial insult to the central nervous system (CNS) most commonly occurs before birth.
- Despite popular belief, hypoxia at birth is not a common cause of CP.
- Physiotherapy is the bedrock of management of CP.
- Gait analysis has enabled surgery to be tailored to the individual child.

Background and incidence

Cerebral palsy is the most common physical disability in childhood.[1] It was originally described by the British 19th-century doctor Little, who later went on to set up the National Orthopaedic Hospital in Stanmore, Middlesex. In the English language literature, CP is still sometimes known as Little's disease while, in Europe, it is more likely to be known as Freud's disease. Before he went on to develop psychotherapy, Sigmund Freud helped to define the patterns of neurological involvement in CP. Freud succeeded in defining a classification system for CP that remains in use to this day and also contributed extensively to the description of various movement disorder syndromes in childhood.[2]

For his part, Little's assertion that CP occurs as a result of 'difficult deliveries' has made life difficult for generations of obstetricians. In contrast, Freud emphasised foetal influences on the pathogenesis of the disease.[3,4] Since then, lawyers acting for bereaved parents have quoted Little and lawyers acting for the beleaguered obstetricians have tried to place the blame for CP along a 'Freudian' path. As will be discussed below, we now know that both mechanisms are important in the development of CP.

CP should be regarded as a collection of disorders with a common theme rather than as a specific disease.

Definition

CEREBRAL PALSY – a chronic neurological disorder of movement and posture, due to a non-progressive defect or lesion of the immature brain.

An overview of management

In the management of CP, the orthopaedic surgeon is but one member of an 'orchestra' and the 'orchestral conductor' is the paediatrician. The management of CP is directed at treating the effects of the neurological lesion rather than the lesion itself.

Developmental and genetic factors are probably responsible in a majority of cases, with 10% due to intrapartum disaster. Except in its mildest forms, CP presents in the first 18 months of life, usually when a child fails to reach its normal motor milestones.

Why is cerebral palsy described as non-progressive?

The term 'non-progressive' serves to distinguish CP from other conditions such as childhood tumours, storage diseases, or Huntington's chorea. Nevertheless, the term is perhaps surprising, given that the child with CP appears to represent a highly dynamic musculoskeletal picture. In fact, damage to the CNS is non-progressive, while the actual disability changes rapidly as the child grows. The immature brain can stage a functional recovery from some early insults through a process known as **neuroplasticity**, but this has limits and once brain tissue is damaged it cannot usually be revived. It has sometimes been suggested that CP merely represents the impact of a cerebrovascular accident (CVA) on a child. There's some truth in this, but the big difference is that a child with CP has to go through its entire growth and development with grossly abnormal forces acting across its bones and joints. Under these conditions, joints dislocate and bones shrink and curve.

Incidence

CP affects about 1 in 500 live births. During the 1950s, it was widely suggested that the incidence of CP would fall. Confidence in advancing obstetric techniques and neonatal care was so high that it seemed likely that the causes of CP would disappear. Unfortunately, this prophecy has only partly been fulfilled. For example, kernicterus (haemolytic disease of the newborn) used to be a significant cause of athetoid CP, but due to the improved management of neonatal jaundice, it is now uncommon. Despite such progress, the overall incidence of CP has changed little. This is in part due to the ability to keep more premature babies alive and in part due to the fact that the majority of cases do not arise from obstetric complications – something that was not fully appreciated in the 1950s.

Figure 8.1
The role of neonatal care

Neonatal intensive care has succeeded in saving the lives of babies who might otherwise have died. In addition, improved management of neonatal jaundice has reduced the incidence of atheoid CP. Unfortunately, other babies who would previously have died now survive, but suffer from severe brain damage. The overall prevalence of CP has remained almost unchanged in the West.

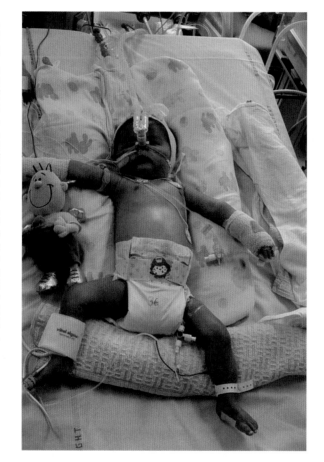

Key points

- CP is not a specific disorder but a collection of disorders with a common theme.
- It is mostly due to developmental and genetic factors with only 10% due to intrapartum problems.
- The neurological damage is non-progressive, but the effect on bones, joints and muscles is not.
- Management must be multi-disciplinary.

Risk factors and classification of cerebral palsy

Risk factors

The initial insult may occur before, during, or after birth.[2]

Prenatal risk factors: placental insufficiency, toxaemia, smoking, drugs, and alcohol. Maternal infection may be responsible, and the mnemonic TORCH reminds us of the likely agents: **To**xoplasmosis, **r**ubella, **C**MV, and **h**erpes simplex. Genetic conditions and failure of normal brain cell migration can also be responsible for CP.

Perinatal risk factors: prematurity, particularly if the birth weight is below 1.5kg. Breech presentation is a risk factor, as are infections such as meningitis and encephalitis. Kernicterus should be an increasingly uncommon cause.

Postnatal risk factors: infection and trauma are most commonly encountered.

Cerebral palsy and hypoxia

There is a popular belief that CP is caused by hypoxia during birth and certainly medico–legal cases often focus on this.[5] Prematurity *per se* does not lead to hypoxia, because pre-term infants are actually better protected against hypoxic insult than term babies. The significance of prematurity is that before about 32 weeks, the blood vessels within the brain are unsupported by connective tissue and are easily damaged or torn by the pressure changes during delivery.

Classification of cerebral palsy

CP may be classified in topographical terms – hemiplegia, diplegia (the most common), or total body affected – or neurological – spastic (exaggerated contraction in response to stretch), athetoid, dystonic (rigidity other than spasticity), or rigid (involuntary sustained muscle contraction not dependent upon stretch). The observed picture depends on the area and extent of brain damage, such as in the cerebral cortex, basal ganglia, or cerebellum. Of these types, spastic CP is by far the most common.

Spasticity is characterised by increased muscle tone and exaggerated spinal reflexes, while athetosis is associated with constant slow, writhing, involuntary movements and is not amenable to surgical intervention.

Ataxia is characterised by poor co-ordination. The child walks with an unbalanced, wide-based gait. Some patients present with a mixed pattern, most commonly spasticity and athetosis. Orthopaedic surgeons are usually concerned with the management of spastic CP.

Cerebral palsy and intelligence

There is a popular belief that CP patients have learning disabilities. However, this is not necessarily the case. About 50% of children with CP will be of normal intelligence or above, and about a quarter go on to lead independent adult lives. One-third will suffer from epilepsy and 25–80% will have speech disorders.

Presentation

CP may not be an obvious diagnosis at birth. Only those with severe CP may lack sucking or blinking reflexes from the start. Later, the persistence of primitive reflexes such as the Moro or the parachute reflex is a significant sign. The persistence of two or more primitive reflexes usually means that the child will be non-ambulatory. On the other hand, a child with mild CP may only present at walking age or even later.

Key points

- Risk factors may be prenatal, perinatal, or postnatal.
- Immature unsupported blood vessels in the brain are easily damaged by pressure changes during premature birth.
- The persistence of primitive reflexes is an indication of possible CP.
- Mild cases may not present until walking age or even later.

Milestones and physical treatment options

Milestones and indicators

Most children learn how to perform specific tasks by a certain age. Some of these tasks have been well documented and are referred to as motor milestones. In cerebral palsy, these motor milestones are likely to be delayed (see Box 8.1 for normal milestones). In addition, there may be tiptoe walking, a clumsy gait, or more unusually, in-toeing. Note that CP is not necessarily symmetrical.

As a rule of thumb, almost all hemiplegic children will walk, whilst only three-quarters of diplegic and less than a quarter of quadriplegic children walk.

Children who by two years can sit will probably go on to walk, but if sitting is only achieved at three years, only about half will walk. Those who can stand by four years will probably accomplish walking. The failure to walk by the time a child is seven years is not a good prognostic sign.

Box 8.1   **Normal milestones in development of motor functions.**

Head up	3 months
Sit unaided	6 months
Crawl	8 months
Pull to stand	10–12 months
Walking	12–15 months

Ambulation

Patients vary in their ability to walk. A simple classification defines community ambulators, household ambulators, therapeutic walkers, and non-walkers, and these can be sub-classified according to the use or otherwise of walking aids. Non-walkers can be further classified in terms of their ability to sit.

CP normally tends to go through three stages:
- **stage one:** dynamic contracture
- **stage two:** muscle contracture
- **stage three:** secondary bone changes (for example, contractures that lead to dislocations and torsional deformity).

Physiotherapy

Physiotherapy is really the bedrock of CP management. In stage one, physiotherapy attempts to prevent the progression of the disease to stage two by stretching and correctly positioning joints. In many cases the parents can be taught to supervise the child's exercises themselves. The prevention of deformity requires regular stretches and a range of movement activities. Splintage may be minimally effective. The true role of the physiotherapist is to attempt to maximise the motor development of the child.

Orthotics

Traditional callipers came to be regarded as a form of stigmatisation. In modern times thermoplastic splints that are more cosmetically acceptable have replaced them. More recently, sophisticated orthotics have been used in combination with medical and surgical procedures. Other treatment options include special seating, nutritional advice, developing communication skills, and the promotion of recreation and sports.

Figure 8.2
Thermoplastic ankle foot orthosis

Modern materials have produced AFOs that are far more lightweight, comfortable and attractive than the traditional and stigmatising callipers of yesteryear. Each AFO is custom made to fit into the child's leg and as the child grows he or she will require new AFOs.

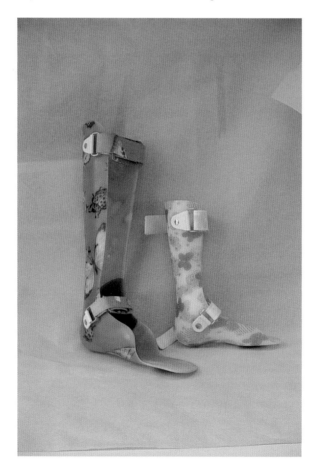

Key points

- Motor milestones are delayed and have some predictive value of future disability.
- Almost all hemiplegic children will be able to walk.
- Those not walking by the age of seven are unlikely to ever do so.
- Physiotherapy is the mainstay of treatment and parents can be taught many of the procedures.

Medical treatments

Botulinum toxin

Commercially available botulinum toxin is being used increasingly in the treatment of CP, as it causes a local relaxation of muscles.[8,9] It does this by blocking transmission at the neuromuscular junction. At the same time as moderating spasticity, there is some evidence that voluntary muscle function also improves. Unfortunately, the body soon makes new neuromuscular junctions and muscle spasm recurs. Reports of a botulinum product being used as a cosmetic agent may sound alarming, but in the context of CP its use is acceptable and the agent is very safe in skilled hands.[10,11]

Method of administration

The toxin can be injected into muscles under general anaesthetic or with sedation. The most commonly injected muscle groups are the hamstrings, the calf, and the hip adductors. The effect lasts for three to six months and injections can then be repeated. Development of an allergy to repeated injections has been described.

Intrathecal baclofen[12]

Baclofen is effective in CP as a muscle relaxant and has gained popularity in the US in the past ten years. Orally, baclofen has unpleasant side effects, but by injecting the drug intrathecally the total dose required can be greatly reduced. Delivery systems involve an intrathecal catheter linked to a reservoir of baclofen implanted into the abdomen. Electronic devices then control a steady flow of the drug into the spinal column where it reduces muscle spasticity. This system, though complex, has the advantage over surgery that it is reversible and the dose can be titrated to the patient's needs. It probably does not help walking diplegics and is mainly used for spastic quadriplegics who can only sit. Serious complications include infection around the spinal cord.

Figure 8.3
Botox injections

Botox injections into key muscle groups affected by spasticity may help to reduce joint contractures. The effects are unlikely to last more than 3–4 months and the injections need to be repeated.

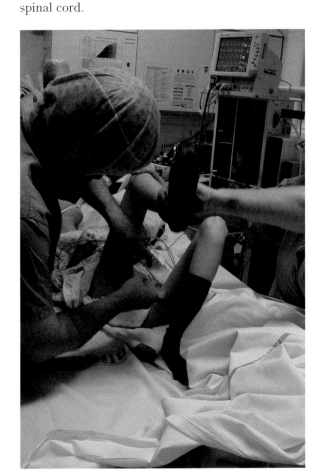

Key points

- Botulinum toxin causes local relaxation of muscles.
- It wears off over 3–6 months but can be repeated.
- Baclofen can help quadriplegics, but must be given intrathecally.
- The delivery system is complex and infection is a serious complication.

The role of orthopaedic surgery

Earlier attempts at surgery for CP patients were disappointing. Procedures were performed in sequence and a feature of this era was that a child would be admitted to hospital at yearly intervals for further surgery. This phenomenon became known as the 'birthday syndrome'.

Each surgical procedure attempted to correct an apparent deformity. For example, the Achilles tendon was often lengthened because it appeared to be tight. The child would then be able to walk on the heels, but it soon became apparent that the hamstrings were tight as the patient started to walk in a crouch. In effect, CP children would spend most of their formative years in a medical institution.

The advent of gait analysis[7]

In the late 1970s, the concept of gait analysis arrived from the US, and this led to a change in the accepted philosophy. Three-dimensional gait analysis coupled with dynamic electromyography and other studies have identified specific abnormal gait patterns. This has led to the development of specific surgical procedures tailored to patients' problems.

Surgery is usually performed in order to enable walking patients to continue walking or to reduce the energy expenditure required to walk. In non-walkers it may help achieve a good sitting position. Comprehensive pre-operative assessment is crucial in selecting the appropriate procedures and the timing of surgery is also of great importance.

In stage two CP, the orthopaedic surgeon can perform tendon-lengthening procedures, and at stage three, osteotomies, joint fusions, and further tendon lengthening can correct bony deformities and dislocations. The timing and scope of these surgical interventions has been much improved by using gait studies.

Selective dorsal root rhizotomy[13]

This procedure involves partially cutting through the sensory nerve roots in the spine to reduce muscle tone in spastic diplegic CP. It is popular in the US, but is little used in the UK. It is not used in the upper limbs and will not correct existing joint contractures. The relaxation achieved is irreversible and it requires extensive surgery that may weaken the spine. Current consensus is that, with careful selection, selective rhizotomy is most suited to the walking child.

Scoliosis

Scoliosis is the most common spinal disorder in CP. Those with quadriplegia are most at risk. Braces and custom-moulded seats allow for better positioning, but neither prevents progression of the curve, which tends to be C-shaped and involves most or the entire spine. Such scoliotic curves can be fixed surgically, but this is a major undertaking.

Upper limb

Few patients are suitable for surgery to the upper limb. Most surgical procedures attempt to place the arm in a more functional position. Orthotic devices are not well-tolerated in the arm.

Key points

- Earlier attempts at surgery resulted in the 'birthday syndrome' of annual procedures.
- Gait analysis and electromyography can identify specific gait patterns.
- Correcting scoliosis is a major surgical undertaking.
- Surgery has little to offer upper-limb problems.

References

1. Rosenbaum P. Cerebral palsy: what parents and doctors want to know. *BMJ* 2003; **326**: 970–4.
2. Accordo PJ. Freud on diplegia. Commentary and translation. *Am J Dis Child* 1982; **136(5)**: 452–6.
3. Lou HC. Hypoxia – haemodynamic pathogenesis of brain lesions in the new born. *Brain Dev* 1994; **16(6)**: 423–31.
4. George MS. Changing nineteenth century views on the origin of cerebral palsy. WJ Little and Sigmund Freud. *J Hist Neuro Sci* 1992; **1**: 29–37.
5. Nelson KB. What proportion of cerebral palsy is related to birth asphyxia? *J Paediatr* 1988; **112**: 572–4.
6. Dear P, Newell S. Establishing probable cause in cerebral palsy. [Letter] *BMJ* 2000; **320**: 1075.
7. Gage J. Gait analysis. An essential tool in the treatment of cerebral palsy. *Clin Orthop* 1993; **288**: 126–34.
8. Cosgrove AP, Corry IS, Graham HK. Botulinum toxin in the management of the lower limb in cerebral palsy. *Develop Med Child Neurol* 1994; **36**: 379–85.
9. Sarioglu B, Serdaruglu G, Tutuncuoglu S, Ozer EA. The use of botulinum toxin A treatment in children with spasticity. Pediatric Neurol 2003 October; **29(4)**: 299–301.
10. Misra VP. The changed image of botulinum toxin. [Editorial] *BMJ* 2002; **325**: 1188.
11. Munchau A, Bhatia KP. Regular review: uses of botulinum toxin injection in medicine today. *BMJ* 2000; **320**: 161–5.
12. Butler C, Cambell S. Evidence of the effects of intrathecal baclofen for spastic and

dystonic cerebral palsy. AACPDM Treatment Outcomes Committee Review Panel. *Dev Med Child Neurol* 2000; **42:** 634–45.

13. Oppenheim WD. Selective posterior rhizotomy for spastic cerebral palsy. A review. *Clin Orthop* 1990; **253:** 20–9.

Chapter Nine

THE ADULT FOOT AND ANKLE

Alison Edwards and Steven Cutts

Problems with the feet can occur in isolation or as part of a multi-system disorder. For example, diabetes and RA are both common causes of foot pathology.

The first priority with any foot problem is to enable the patient to be able to walk without pain. The ability to wear normal footwear is also desirable. However, in practice, many operations are performed for cosmetic reasons. Most foot problems can be managed using conservative measures such as orthotics, splintage, or footwear modifications. Common problems are outlined in Box 9.1. Some of these are discussed in detail in this chapter.

Box 9.1 **Common foot problems**

Hallux valgus	Hallux rigidus
Plantar fasciitis	Achilles tendinitis or rupture
Lesser toe deformities	Morton's neuroma
Tibialis posterior dysfunction	Ankle or subtalar arthritis
Diabetic feet	Gout

Hallux valgus in the adult

Adult hallux valgus is one of the most common foot deformities. It is classically seen in women between 50 and 70 years of age, and in about two-thirds of cases there is a positive family history. It is usually bilateral, but it may be more severe on one side than the other. In most cases hallux valgus is not painful, except when tight-fitting shoes cause inflammation.

The nature of the hallux valgus deformity

In hallux valgus the big toe deviates laterally. The medial border of the metatarso-phalangeal (MTP) joint of the big toe becomes more prominent and the overlying soft tissues start to swell. Later, bony osteophytes may appear around the joint. All these factors lead to a prominent MTP joint that rubs against footwear and is also unsightly. The medial swelling constitutes a **bunion** and the overlying skin may become inflamed and tender. Once the MTP deformity exceeds about 30 degrees, the pull of the long flexor tendons exacerbates the angle to the point where it becomes irreversible. In many cases, an overriding second toe soon develops.

The deformity is often more obvious when the patient stands up. When requesting X-rays in hallux valgus, always specify that the patient must be **weight bearing**.

Figure 9.1
Hallux Valgus

Hallux valgus in a young woman with an overriding second toe. The first MTP joint is prominent on the medial side.

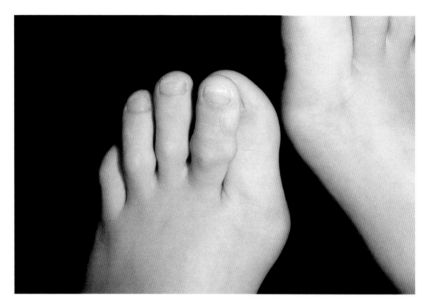

The role of shoes

Special orthopaedic shoes have been developed for hallux valgus, with a wide, deep toe-box. Unfortunately, these shoes are never pretty and always out of fashion. This may not be a concern for many elderly patients, who are simply grateful for special footwear, but younger patients will often ask for surgery to improve the cosmetic appearance of their feet. Being able to fit into fashionable shoes is also a key issue for the younger patient. With these thoughts in mind, remember that it's important to ask the patient exactly what bothers them about the bunion. The presence of hallux valgus does not in itself require active treatment.

Hallux valgus in adolescence

Teenagers form a specific subgroup of hallux valgus patients that deserve special attention. Pain is not a common complaint, but, as mentioned, young patients are more likely to be bothered by the cosmetic appearance of their feet. There is often a family history of the condition and the patient is likely to be accompanied by a parent who wishes to see the problem corrected.

This issue is discussed in more depth in Chapter 6.

Hallux valgus in older people

Older people are more likely to be concerned by pain than by cosmesis. Secondary OA is often present, so many surgeons treat elderly patients with joint fusion.

Surgical procedures

The choice of surgical procedure will depend upon the degree of deformity, where the deformity lies, whether it can be passively corrected, the patient's age, and the surgeon's preferred technique. When counselling a patient for possible surgery it is important to explain that post-operative pain may be experienced for up to six months. Most procedures have a success rate of about 85%. Inevitably, some patients end up having repeat surgery. Many types of operation require patients to wear a plaster slipper for six weeks and some require a wire to be inserted through the toe for up to six weeks.

Hallux rigidus

The big toe is capable of about 70 degrees of dorsiflexion. This is essential to normal walking and is maximal just as the foot clears the ground for the next stride. In hallux rigidus, there is painful restriction of movement of the big toe, which is often worse in the mornings. A long first metatarsal may predispose to this condition, but other causes include inflammatory arthritis or occupational stresses. Professional footballers often develop hallux rigidus from the trauma of repeated kicking. In the elderly it is often associated with gout. An osteophyte on the superior aspect of the joint may be responsible for the pain or restriction in movement. In younger adults there may be a history of injury or osteochondritis dissecans.

Treatment

Some patients respond to a shoe with a rocker-bottom sole. This enables the foot to take off without dorsiflexion of the toe. Simple painkillers may also help. Where symptoms are not controlled by conservative measures, surgery might be considered. Excision of a dorsal osteophyte may be all that is needed, but osteotomy, arthrodesis, and arthroplasty are other possibilities. Of these, arthrodesis (fusion) is probably the most reliable. Silicone MTP joint replacements have been tried but with disappointing results.

Plantar fasciitis

Plantar fasciitis causes pain in the sole or heel of the foot and is more common in the 40–65 age-group. Plantar fasciitis has also been termed 'policeman's heel'. It is thought to be a chronic injury (reparative process) and the pain is typically worse when the patient first gets out of bed. One theory is that as the patient lies in bed at night, their foot drops down into plantar flexion and the planter fascia slightly shrinks. In the morning, as the patient walks around again, the fascia is stretched out to length and this causes the pain. For this reason, some patients benefit from night splints that hold the foot in dorsiflexion (i.e. at a right angle) through the night.[1]

Plantar fasciitis may also be associated with other inflammatory disorders but mostly occurs with overuse or after recent weight gain. Symptoms may be eased by NSAIDs, insoles, wearing flat shoes, and steroid injections. Physiotherapy can stretch the tight Achilles tendon complex often found in this condition. A calcaneal spur seen on X-ray is rarely of any significance. Surgery is hardly ever necessary. Other causes of heel pain, such as infection, tumours, arthropathies, and stress fractures, should be considered if the patient is not responding to treatment.

Achilles tendinitis

Achilles tendinitis may be due to a painful inflammation of the tendon sheath, degenerative changes within the tendon, or a combination of both. The hypovascular region of the tendon, about 4–6cm proximal to its insertion, is most prone to overuse repetitive injury, so it is common in runners, especially if they run on roads.

Treatment requires careful attention to training regimes, appropriate footwear, and physiotherapy. Some sports physicians use steroid injections, but this may be associated with subsequent rupture. Occasionally, surgical exploration and excision of inflamed tissue proves successful.

Achilles tendon rupture[2]

Rupture of the Achilles tendon is a common and serious problem. It often occurs when patients in their 30s and 40s attempt a return to sport after years of a sedentary existence. Patients may report hearing an audible 'pop' when leaping up to catch or hit a ball. If they are playing a team game, patients may think they have been kicked in the back of the ankle by another player. Predisposing factors include oral steroids and diabetes.

The diagnosis should be straightforward, based on the history and physical signs, but about 25% of cases are missed. There is usually a palpable gap in the tendon that can be easily felt about 2–6cms proximal to its insertion. Simmond's test is helpful in diagnosis – the calf is squeezed whilst the foot hangs over the edge of the couch. If the tendon is intact, the ankle will plantar flex.

Biographical note
Simmond's test is named after a British twentieth-century orthopaedic surgeon. However, the term 'Thompson's test' is used interchangeably after the American surgeon.

Whilst sitting in a chair, a patient with a ruptured Achilles tendon is still able to actively plantar flex the ankle by using the long flexors of the toes. This ability can be mistakenly interpreted as meaning the Achilles tendon is intact. The key test is to ask the patient to stand on tip-toe on one leg. If the Achilles tendon is ruptured, standing on tip-toe is impossible.

Treatment

Achilles tendon rupture can be treated conservatively or with surgery. With conservative treatment, the leg is put in a plaster cast in full plantar flexion. A plaster is usually required for six to eight weeks. Every three to four weeks the cast is changed and the degree of flexion decreased until after about three changes, the foot is back into a normal position. Most patients respond well and a heel raise is often recommended for two to three months after removal of the cast. Sport should be avoided for up to a year. There is a 10–15% chance of re-rupture after conservative management.

Surgical treatment

The ends of the ruptured tendon can be sutured together in an open procedure. The leg is then placed in a plaster cast as in conservative management. There is a debate about which treatment is best. Surgery carries a small risk of deep infection, but there is a less than 5% risk of re-rupture and performance athletes do better in competitive sport after surgery than after conservative management. In the UK, most orthopaedic surgeons would only consider surgery in younger patients who hope to return to competitive sport.

Sometimes the diagnosis is only made many weeks or months after the event. In these circumstances it is impossible to treat a ruptured Achilles tendon in a plaster cast. Surgical reconstruction may be needed in the younger, active patient, but older patients may cope with a brace.

Toe deformities

Most patients present because the deformed toes are rubbing against footwear and causing painful corns, either on the sole of the foot or on the dorsal surface of the interphalangeal (IP) joints. Most patients put up with minor deformities or may be helped by shoes with a wider box toe and soft leather uppers. Severe cases may justify surgery to the tendons or even joint fusion.

Claw toes

In claw toes, the IP joints are flexed and the MTP joints extended. They are usually idiopathic but may be associated with neurological problems. Claw toes are also found in rheumatoid feet and in high-arched feet.

Hammer toes

With hammer toes, the proximal joint is flexed and the distal joint extended. It often affects the second toe. Painful callosities can occur and surgical correction can be offered if symptoms are troublesome.

Mallet toe

In a mallet toe, the distal IP joint is flexed. Symptomatic cases may benefit from surgery.

Over-riding fifth toes

Over-riding fifth toes are often a congenital deformity and can be corrected by surgery if necessary.

Morton's neuroma

Morton's neuroma causes a hypersensitive area in the forefoot, due to entrapment and irritation of one of the interdigital nerves. Tenderness is maximal in one of the spaces between the metatarsals, most commonly the third and fourth, often with paraesthesiae and numbness in the affected toes. Squeezing the forefoot exacerbates the pain, so tight-fitting shoes make the problem worse. The condition is common in mature, fashion-conscious women. The diagnosis can be confirmed by injecting local anaesthetic around the nerve. Some surgeons recommend a broader fitting shoe or a metatarsal bar to unload the forefoot, but this may not be acceptable to the patient. In persistent cases surgery is usually effective. Potential complications are end-stump neuroma and recurrence.

Biographical note

Thomas George Morton *(1835–1903), highly celebrated American Civil War Surgeon. Born 1835 in Philadelphia – died 1903 from cholera. Co-founder of The Hospital for Nervous Diseases. Best remembered today for his descriptions of Morton's metatarsalgia and also Morton's neuroma.*

Tarsal tunnel syndrome

Tarsal tunnel syndrome is similar to carpal tunnel syndrome and patients with posterior tibial nerve compression get symptoms of pain and paraesthesiae in the feet. As in the hand, the symptoms are worse at night. The medial part of the foot is affected. The problem is compression of the posterior tibial nerve in the fibro-osseous tunnel behind the medial malleolus. Tinel's sign (tingling along the distribution of the nerve when it is tapped) may be present, with numbness of the sole. Nerve conduction studies may distinguish it from referred pain from a herniated lumbar disc.

NSAIDs, orthotics, and injections may be helpful. If they are not, and the diagnosis is clear, decompression produces improvement in 75% of cases.

Biographical note
Jules Tinel, *French neurologist (1879–1952), realised that tapping over an area of damaged or regenerating nerve caused tingling in that nerve. Tinel was head of the neurological centre at Mans in World War I and an active member of the French resistance in World War II. Captured and imprisoned by the Nazis, he survived and went back into practice but died of heart failure in 1952.*

Tibialis posterior dysfunction

After the Achilles tendon, tibialis posterior is the second strongest tendon in the body. Together with **peroneus longus** (which descends from the lateral side) it forms a tendinous sling that holds up the arches in the foot. If the tibialis posterior tendon ruptures, the arches of the foot gradually collapse and the patient develops a planovalgus foot.

Figure 9.2
'Too many toes sign'

There are more toes visible laterally on the left side than on then right. This is left-sided planovalgus foot secondary to ruptured tibialis posterior tendon.

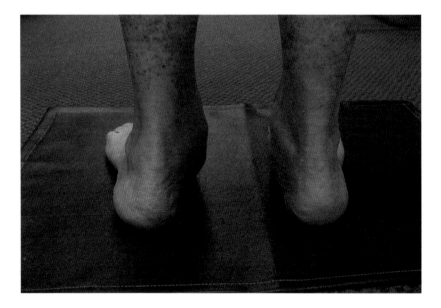

However, there are less spectacular ailments that can affect the tibialis posterior than rupture. Tibialis posterior tendon dysfunction ranges from mild tendinitis to overt rupture of the tendon leading to an acquired flat foot deformity in the older patient. Predisposing factors for frank rupture include hypertension, obesity, diabetes, inflammatory arthropathies, and previous foot surgery. The condition tends to be under-diagnosed.

In the early stages of tibialis posterior tendinitis, swelling and pain are localised behind the medial malleolus. The patient is able to stand on tip-toe, but with pain, and the medial foot arch is intact. As the problem progresses, the tendon may stretch or rupture and a flexible flat foot deformity develops. This may later become a rigid flat foot due to mid- and hindfoot degenerative arthritis. Early on, a medial arch support, NSAIDs, and physiotherapy may settle things down. With a painful, rigid flat foot, a triple arthrodesis of the hindfoot may be needed.

Figure 9.3
Flat right foot

This patient has a planovalgus right foot, again secondary to an incompetent tibialis posterior tendon. The arches have completely disappeared.

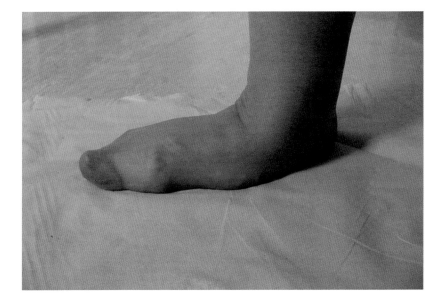

Ankle and subtalar arthritis

RA and other inflammatory arthritides is more common. Approximately 20–40% of patients get OA after an ankle fracture and its incidence, as with any fracture, is increased in more severe injuries. Classically, the subtalar joint produces pain when walking on uneven ground. Hindfoot arthritis not uncommonly leads to a valgus deformity. The use of orthoses can help improve pain.

One common surgical solution to hindfoot arthritis is joint fusion, which provides a reliable form of pain relief. Unfortunately, joint fusion puts extra stress on adjacent joints and the patient may then develop further arthritis elsewhere in the foot. For this reason, many surgeons prefer to fuse joints in older patients who may not do as much walking.

Hindfoot arthritis in a younger patient is more of a challenge. These patients have a greater life expectancy and they tend to average more miles per year. Arthroscopic debridement is sometimes used in mild-to-moderate OA of the ankle.

Ankle replacement is now possible but is still regarded as a novel procedure. The long-term results are improving.[3] Part of the problem with an ankle replacement is how to salvage it when it fails. Replacing the ankle joint is usually reserved for non-obese patients who are 'low demand', e.g. patients with RA.

Only a minority of orthopaedic surgeons have any experience in ankle replacements and many of these have only done a modest number. Doubtless, in the future, experience in the technique will improve.

References

1. Berlet GC, Anderson RB, Davis H, Kiebzak EM. A prospective trial of night splinting in the treatment of recalcitrant plantar fasciitis: the Ankle Dorsiflexion Dynasplint. *Orthopedics* 2002; **25(11):** 1273–5.

2. Cohen RS, Balcom TA. Current treatment options for ankle injuries: lateral ankle sprain, Achilles tendonitis and Achilles rupture. *Curr Sports Med Rep* 2003; **2(5):** 251–4.

3. Anderson T, Montgomery F, Carlsson A. Uncemented STAR total ankle prosthesis. Three to eight-year follow-up of fifty-one consecutive ankles. *J Bone Joint Surg Am* 2003; **85-A(7):** 1321–9.

Chapter Ten

THE CERVICAL SPINE

Alison Edwards and Steven Cutts

Cervical spondylosis

A high proportion of people will experience neck pain at some time in their life, but only a few will go on to develop serious neurological problems.

The term 'spondylosis' covers a collection of symptomatic degenerative changes that can occur throughout the spine. Many degenerative changes are merely manifestations of normal age-related wear rather than of a disease. Consequently, cervical spondylosis is a difficult label to attach to someone presenting with characteristic symptoms.

Cervical spondylosis is more common in men than women. Typically, symptoms begin in the 50–60-year-old age group. In the cervical spine, C5/6 is the most commonly affected joint. Remember that 60% of rotational movement in the neck is at C1/C2 and that most flexion occurs at C5/6. *Lateral flexion* is the first movement to be lost in cervical spondylosis. Neck pain may radiate up to the occiput and also down to the shoulders and arms, but referred neck pain does not usually go below the elbow. Pain radiating below the elbow suggests nerve root pain or peripheral nerve entrapment.

Neck pain is usually self-limiting. One study showed that up to 78% of cervical neck pain resolves or improves within three months. Special imaging is rarely necessary early on. Patients who accept minor chronic changes and live with them are likely to do well. Other patients do not accept the symptoms and demand a solution. Patient education is important to help them modify their work and other activities to avoid actions that provoke symptoms.

Surgical cervical fusion is reserved for specific indications. Once this is accomplished, stress on the joints above and below the fused joint increases and this can accelerate degeneration of these joints. Broadly speaking, hard and soft collars are not recommended for the treatment of the degenerate spine. They are not greatly beneficial and make the patient reluctant to exercise the neck, encouraging stiffness.

Whiplash

Does whiplash accelerate spondylosis?

Many people involved in traffic accidents claim compensation for whiplash injuries. However, the influence of whiplash on the progression of spondylotic disease is controversial. Some surgeons believe that many patients exaggerate their whiplash symptoms to obtain financial compensation for injury. It is often pointed out that whiplash is rarely seen in countries where the law does not allow for financial compensation.

Discogenic pain

Discogenic pain may begin insidiously and may be present without neurological abnormalities. The pain is usually exacerbated by movement. There is limited range of movement, sometimes with crepitus. No neurological signs are usually detectable. In these cases treatment is usually conservative; i.e. simple painkillers, physiotherapy.

Risk factors for spondylotic change

- smoking
- excessive driving
- frequent lifting
- advancing age
- family history

Assessment of cervical radiculopathy

The radical here is the spinal nerve root leaving the spinal cord and making its way to the neck or arm via the exit foramina. These nerve roots may be irritated or even compressed during this journey. Classically this may occur due to a slipped disc in the neck although a narrow exit foraminum (due to cervical osteophytes) may have the same effect. Once this happens, the patient will notice altered sensation in the distribution of that nerve root.

The symptoms include neck, shoulder, and arm pain with paraesthesiae and numbness, radiating in a dermatomal pattern. Movement may exacerbate the pain. The arm pain is usually worse than the neck pain. Tilting the head to one side may relieve the arm pain. Radiculopathy may involve more than one root. The root most commonly affected is C7, followed by C6, but it may be difficult to determine the level from which symptoms arise, because of overlap between dermatomal segments. There may also be muscle weakness in a myotomal pattern.

Reflexes may also be suppressed in the elbow and forearm.

There are four main reasons why a nerve root can be painful:

1. disc herniation
2. pressure on the nerve from chondro-osseous spurs from the uncovertebral joint
3. pressure on the nerve due to narrowing of the nerve foramen when disc height is lost
4. inflammation around the nerve root.

Patients with cervical radiculopathy due to a disc herniation are generally younger than those with spondylosis and usually give an acute history. Neurological examination is obviously the key to reaching an accurate diagnosis and, within this, detecting a motor radiculopathy with an absent reflex and corresponding loss of a myotomal level would indicate a more severe root entrapment. Plain X-rays are frequently normal.

Investigations

When assessing patients with suspected cervical radiculopathy, consider other causes, including pathology in the shoulder, chest, and arms. The differential diagnosis includes spinal and extra spinal tumours (such as Pancoast tumour, brachial plexus lesions, thoracic outlet syndrome), shoulder conditions (such as frozen shoulder, subacromial impingement), and peripheral nerve entrapment (such as carpal tunnel syndrome).

Plain X-rays are a good starting point, but appearances often do not correlate with the patient's clinical condition. Severe spondylotic changes on an X-ray may be a coincidental finding. Anteroposterior, lateral, and flexion/extension views are needed.

X-ray changes in cervical spondylosis are similar to those of ageing. On plain X-ray, 40% of 50-year-olds and 70% of 70-year-olds have degenerative changes of the cervical spine. Unless these are symptomatic, they should not be labelled as cervical spondylosis.

MRI scans are excellent for showing soft tissue detail but can still mislead. On MRI, a quarter of asymptomatic patients over 40 years old are found to have a herniated disc, with or without stenosis of the nerve root foramen.

Treatment of cervical radiculopathy

For mild cases, conservative treatments include NSAIDs, heat, a soft

Figure 10.1
Cervical spine illustration

This sagittal MRI scan shows the spinal cord being compressed by a dramatic abnormality in the mid-cervical region. MRI enables the visualisation of the discs, ligaments and even the structure of the hind brain and spinal cord, in addition to the bones.

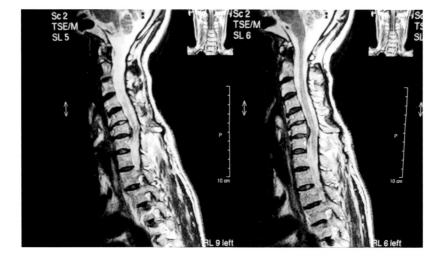

collar, physiotherapy, and referral to a pain clinic. Controversy plagues all forms of treatment, including complementary therapies. It may take up to six months for symptoms to resolve.

Indications for GP referral:

- Radiculitis alone – if not resolving by six weeks.
- Radiculitis and sensory or motor radiculopathy – refer straight away to spinal service for assessment.
- Myelopathy – refer straight away.

Surgery

If conservative management fails, the surgical options include discectomy, foraminal decompression, laminectomy, and fusion. This kind of surgery has to be done by a career spinal surgeon. Where arm pain is severe, and the patient is prepared to accept the possibility of being made worse, then surgery is usually offered. Motor deficits are unlikely to resolve, even with surgery, which also carries a risk of iatrogenic nerve injury.

Cervical myelopathy

Myelopathy is usually due to anterior cord compression because of spondylotic changes. Signs include motor weakness, gait problems, and spasticity, and there is often a confusing mixture of upper and lower motor neurone findings. Lower motor neurone findings usually occur at the level of compression and upper motor neurone signs below this. It is usually the latter that are more easily recognised in the clinical examination.

Table 10.1   **Assessing the level of radiculopathy**

Level	Root	Pain	Paraesthesiae	Weakness	Reflex
C3/4	C4	neck, shoulder	lateral neck, shoulder	scapular muscles	–
C4/5	C5	shoulder, upper arm, deltoid	regimental badge	deltoid, biceps	biceps
C5/6	C6	neck, biceps, radial forearm, dorsum of hand between thumb and middle finger	radial forearm	wrist extensors, biceps	biceps, brachio-radialis
C6/7	C7	back of shoulder, triceps, posterior forearm, middle finger	middle finger	triceps, wrist flexors	triceps
C7/8	C8	ring and little fingers	ulnar hand	fingers flexed, interossei	–
C8/T1	T1	medial forearm	ulnar forearm	interossei	–

Cervical stenosis can be congenital or acquired; for example, as a result of posterior vertebral osteophytes, subluxing vertebra, or facet joint hypertrophy. Cord ischaemia may result from interruption of the blood supply. Later secondary changes in the spinal cord include distortion of cord tissue and demyelination of white matter.

More than 70% of patients with myelopathy will get progressively worse, but it is difficult to predict those who will deteriorate. Patients may present with a minor deficit without recent progression or with severe disability with relentless progression. More often, the onset is gradual, as the spondylosis gradually causes cervical stenosis and cord compromise.

Occasionally, onset is sudden due to acute disc herniation in an already narrow spinal canal. These patients with cervical stenosis in addition to impending or actual cervical myelopathy are also at risk of spinal cord injury with minimal traumatic neck extension. This causes anterior spinal cord syndrome. Anterior cord damage tends to affect legs more than the arms. Propioception is not affected. The diagnosis is largely based on history and physical examination.

Symptoms and signs

- patients may fall frequently
- they experience burning, stinging pain, and Lhermitte's phenomenon – an electric shock pain down the arm when they flex the neck
- nerve root symptoms are present
- urinary disturbance occurs at a late stage
- motor weakness is generally more pronounced in the arms
- patients may have an ataxic, broad-based, shuffling gait
- involvement of legs with spasticity is a bad sign

Upper motor neurone findings include hyperreflexia, Hoffman's sign, Babinski's sign, the finger escape sign (little finger abduction because of weak intrinsics), and ankle clonus. Lower motor neurone signs in the upper limb root cause sensory and motor impairment. The pattern may be confusing.

Cervical myelopathy signs

LHERMITTE'S PHENOMENON – an electric shock pain down the arm on flexing the neck.

HOFFMAN'S SIGN – by flicking the middle finger DIPJ into extension, there is a reflex flexion of the thumb and index fingers.

BABINSKI'S SIGN – upward (extensor) movement of the big toe on stroking sole of the foot.

Treatment

In non-progressive mild disease, a semi-rigid orthosis is used and regular review is indicated. The patient or their carers should be educated about which symptoms to look out for and when to seek urgent medical attention. Surgery is indicated when there is difficulty walking, relentlessly progressive disease, or if MRI shows severe compression. The aims are decompression and maintenance of spinal stability. Patients are usually counselled that surgery is performed to prevent further progression and improve pain. The extent of motor recovery is unpredictable.

Rheumatoid arthritis of the cervical spine

Rheumatoid arthritis (RA) is the most common inflammatory arthritis, affecting about 1% of the population and 5% of people over 70. The cervical spine is often badly affected. Joint damage in RA is secondary to the synovitis. The rheumatoid inflammatory tissue (pannus) can cause spondylodiscitis and weaken the ligaments around the neck.

Involvement of the cervical spine is the most life-threatening and disabling manifestation of the disease. Some studies suggest the cervical spine is involved in up to 88% of patients with RA. This tends to happen early in the disease. Although RA is more common in women, cervical spine subluxations are more likely in men. Because intubation can be hazardous, patients with RA have cervical spine X-rays before undergoing GA. Their spinal cord may also be more sensitive to hypotensive ischaemia.

Signs

In addition to neck pain, patients may experience occipital headaches, peripheral neurological symptoms, and Lhermitte's sign. Urinary incontinence or retention may be the first sign. Some patients present with vertebro-basilar insufficiency with vertigo, tinnitus, dysphagia, visual disturbances, or loss of equilibrium. Signs of radiculopathy or myelopathy may be present; up to 10% of patients with RA die this way.

MRI – normally requested by a spinal surgeon – is excellent for detecting soft tissue changes in the neck. Unlike plain X-ray, it will distinguish cord compression by pannus from compression due to vertebral malalignment.

Treatment

The aim of treatment is to prevent the onset of neurological deficit. Disease-modifying agents may prevent progression. A soft collar may help relieve symptoms but has not been shown to prevent progression towards malalignment and cord compression. NSAIDs and trigger-point injections may provide pain relief.

TENS machines and heat massage seem to help, but there is no hard evidence to support their use. Regular monitoring by plain X-ray and if necessary MRI is an important part of non-operative management.

Indications for surgery are:

- impending or actual neurology with instability
- vertebral artery compromise
- intractable pain.

Thoracic outlet syndrome

Thoracic outlet syndrome is a complex of signs and symptoms caused by the compression of neurovascular structures in the thoracic outlet. Trauma may be implicated as a precipitant in up to 60% of cases. Young to middle-aged women are most often affected, with a male to female ratio of 1:4. Obesity and the presence of large breasts are aggravating factors.

The symptoms of thoracic outlet syndrome may be similar to those of cervical spondylosis or ulnar nerve compression at the elbow, combined with neck pain and paraesthesiae that increases with overhead activities. Between 90–95% of patients have paraesthesiae. Many report colour changes, weakness, and fatigability.

In order of frequency, the structures involved are the brachial plexus, subclavian vein, and subclavian artery. Most patients report neurological symptoms. The causes are: cervical ribs or abnormalities of the first rib; anterior scalene muscle constriction or abnormal insertion; abnormal fibrous bands; or the head of the sternomastoid muscle compressing the lateral cord of the brachial plexus.

Assessment

X-rays are indicated to look for causes such as bony cervical ribs or first rib anomalies, or Pancoast tumour. MRI may be useful and EMG studies can help to rule out other peripheral nerve entrapment neuropathies.

Physical signs are neurological and/or vascular. In severe cases the entire brachial plexus may be involved. Venous signs are congestion, swelling and distended veins. Arterial signs are bruits, splinter haemorrhages, and coldness. One of the most well-known tests for thoracic outlet syndrome is Adson's manoeuvre – the symptoms are reproduced when the head is hyper-extended and turned towards the affected side. Obliteration of the pulse with the arm in various positions is not a reliable test, since it may be positive in people with no symptoms.

When sinister causes have been ruled out, treatment options include physiotherapy with stretching of the scalene muscles and postural training, TENS machines, baclofen, and modification of activities.

Surgery is reserved for refractory symptoms or where a mechanical cause has been identified. After surgery, 70–80% of patients report improvement in symptoms, but only 20–30% are truly asymptomatic.

References

1.   Boyce RH, Wang JC. Evaluation of neck pain, radiculopathy and myelopathy, imaging conservative treatment and surgical indications. *American Academy of Orthopaedic Surgeons Instructional Course Lectures* 2003; **52:** 489–95.

2.   Solomon L, Warwick D, Nayagam S. The neck. In: *Apley's System of Orthopaedics and Fractures*. [8th edition.] New York: OUP-USA, 2001; 357–69.

Chapter Eleven

THE SHOULDER AND ELBOW

Steven Cutts, Alison Edwards, and Darren Clarke

The origins of shoulder pain

The most common presenting complaint in shoulder patients is pain, which can originate from a variety of sources, including the shoulder joint itself and the acromioclavicular joint. Pain may also be referred to the shoulder from elsewhere. True shoulder pain is felt around the shoulder, usually radiating down the arm to the level of deltoid insertion. It can also spread out along the radial border of the forearm. Radiation to the hand is unusual, but when this occurs it is to the thenar eminence. Pain reaching as far as the fingers is more likely to be nerve root pain, commonly from the 6th, 7th, and 8th cervical nerves.

Thoracic outlet pain radiates to the chest, axilla, and the ulna side of the forearm. The pain of cervical spondylosis has a variable radiation depending on the level involved but often goes up to the occiput and down to the supraclavicular fossae and upper arms.

Pain from the diaphragm and gall bladder can be referred to the shoulder and cardiac pain can be felt in either shoulder.

The shoulder history

A history of injury may point to a specific diagnosis. A sudden violent force suggests dislocation or fracture, whereas a moderate injury may cause a rotator cuff tear or subluxation.

If there is no specific injury and the pain is of slow onset, then a more likely diagnosis would be impingement, frozen shoulder, or arthritis. Night pain is often a feature of shoulder disorders, especially where there is an inflammatory component. Patients may be unable to lie on the affected side.

Certain activities can provoke particular types of shoulder pain. Window cleaners get rotator cuff pain, whereas tennis players are more likely to have impingement.

Systemic conditions and shoulder pathology

Some systemic conditions predispose to shoulder pathology. For example, the diabetic patient is at increased risk of frozen shoulder. **Sickle cell disease** predisposes to avascular necrosis of the humerus. **Ehlers–Danlos syndrome** (which causes all ligaments to be very lax) predisposes to subluxation and/or dislocation.

Examination

When examining a limb, it's always sensible to start by examining the normal side and then to compare this to the bad side. It's also worth noting the position or activities that make the pain worse. If the pain is worse in adduction, then it may arise from the acromioclavicular joint, whereas pain that worsens on reaching upwards suggests a problem with the rotator cuff. If the pain radiates down the arm and into the hand, a neurological examination should be carried out.

Investigations in shoulder injury

No single investigation provides a certain diagnosis. Plain X-rays are useful as an initial investigation, but they do not directly reveal information about the soft tissues. Arthrography can be useful in adhesive capsulitis (frozen shoulder), but it is expensive and uncomfortable for the patient. In many centres it is regarded as an historical investigation.

An MRI scan of the shoulder is regarded as the investigation of choice by many specialists. It is good at detecting full thickness cuff tears. Contrast MRI arthrography can give even more information. But even MRI has limitations – for example, MRI may not show any abnormality at all in frozen shoulder even though the patient is quite grossly disabled.

Ultrasound is useful for looking at rotator cuff tears and is cheap and readily available. But ultrasound is a real-time, operator-dependent investigation and requires a patient with a mobile shoulder.

Frozen shoulder

The term 'frozen shoulder' was first coined by Codman in 1934.[1] Nearly seventy years later, there is still disagreement as to the cause of the condition and its exact definition. Synonyms for frozen shoulder include 'adhesive capsulitis' and 'check rein syndrome'.

Frozen shoulder is a common condition producing a stiff, painful shoulder. The onset is usually insidious, with middle-aged and elderly people forming the bulk of the patients (peak age is 56 years). It is equally common in men and women and may affect the left or the right side.

As the term suggests, the patient develops an increasingly stiff and painful shoulder. All shoulder movements are restricted, particularly abduction and external rotation. Pain is felt over the insertion of the deltoid muscle and is often especially severe at night. There is a global loss of both active and passive movement in the shoulder. The passive range of external rotation is less than 50% of the unaffected side and there may be some disuse wasting of the deltoid muscle.

Who gets frozen shoulder?

Diabetics are prone to developing frozen shoulder (10–20% risk). As 42% of bilateral frozen shoulder patients have diabetes, it is reasonable to investigate for this if a patient presents with bilateral frozen shoulder. Additionally, 18% of patients with frozen shoulder have Dupuytren's disease in the hands.

Leaving the arm in a sling for a protracted period of time may cause a frozen shoulder. For example, there is an association between Colles' fracture and the development of frozen shoulder.

Box 11.1   **Associated risk factors for frozen shoulder**
- diabetes
- Dupuytren's disease
- hyperlipidaemia
- hyperthyroidism
- cardiac disease
- hemiplegia
- recent neurosurgery
- phenobarbitone treatment

Natural history of frozen shoulder

Classically, the condition will progress through three phases:
1. pain
2. stiffening
3. thawing.

Many authorities claim that even without treatment there will be spontaneous resolution within 18 months to two years. However, it is not uncommon to come across patients who would dispute this!

Aetiology of frozen shoulder

The aetiology of frozen shoulder is quite fascinating. It appears to be a form of fibromatosis.[2] Once a patient develops one form of fibromatosis, he or she is more likely to develop a second.

The term 'adhesive capsulitis' is a recognised synonym for frozen shoulder. However, this term is misleading, since there is no evidence of inflammatory change in a frozen shoulder and adhesions do not occur. Instead, the ligament between the coracoid process and the humerus is affected by fibromatosis. As in Dupuytren's disease, this leads to a contracture of the ligament. The restricted external rotation that is the hallmark of frozen shoulder is explained by corcohumeral ligament shortening. It has also inspired the other synonym, 'check rein syndrome'.

However, with the exception of frozen shoulder, all of these condi-

---

Box 11.2   **Different forms of fibromatosis**

- frozen shoulder
- Dupuytren's disease in the hand
- Ledderhose disease in the sole of the foot
- Peyronie's disease in the penis

---

tions are virtually pain-free at rest. In addition, other forms of fibromatosis never spontaneously resolve. This would suggest that the pathological process in frozen shoulder is more complex than simple fibromatosis.

Diagnostic accuracy

Joint stiffness is a feature of many conditions in orthopaedics and this is particularly true of the shoulder. For example, rotator cuff tears and glenohumeral arthritis may cause stiffness and pain in the joint. However, if a patient presents with a painful shoulder and gross limitation of passive external rotation, there are only three differentials:

1. frozen shoulder
2. glenohumeral osteoarthritis
3. locked posterior dislocation.

Of these three, locked posterior dislocation is incredibly rare. Osteoarthritis of the shoulder is quite common in older people and may well co-exist with frozen shoulder.

Investigations in frozen shoulder
Plain X-ray
There are no specific changes on plain X-ray. There may be mild disuse osteopaenia. Because of the age group affected, there may also be radiological signs of other shoulder pathology, but this is coincidental. Plain X-rays are useful for eliminating glenohumeral osteoarthritis and locked posterior dislocation.

MRI scan
MRI may show thickening of the shoulder capsule, but again, MRI is not diagnostic in frozen shoulder.

Blood tests
Blood tests are unhelpful in frozen shoulder. For example, HLA-B27, ESR, CRP, FBC are all normal in this condition.

Diagnostic arthroscopy
Arthroscopy is diagnostic in frozen shoulder. Biopsy of the affected tissue reveals a histological picture almost identical to Dupuytren's contracture in the hand. Synovitis is another feature of frozen shoulder on arthroscopy. This may in part explain why the condition is painful.

Arthroscopy is also useful for assessing the presence of other pathology within the joint, such as a rotator cuff tear. If the patient has given full consent in advance, it is possible to proceed to surgical release of the contracture in the same procedure.

Arthrogram
Injection of contrast media into the shoulder joint reveals characteristic reduction in joint volume with obliteration of the subscapularis bursa. However, an arthrogram is in some respects an historical investigation.

Treatment
The treatment of a self-limiting condition is usually successful. However, more active patients are unlikely to tolerate the protracted pain and disability brought on by the disease. Recovery can be much accelerated by the following:

Physiotherapy

Many patients respond well to physiotherapy.

Steroid injection

This often seems to help. The orthopaedic literature is divided as to whether such injections alter the speed of recovery.

Manipulation under anaesthesia

MUA is the most predictable treatment for frozen shoulder:

- 75% of patients achieve a near normal range of movement after MUA
- 79% experience a relief of pain
- 75% return to work within nine weeks.

It is reasonable to perform an MUA on diabetic patients, but they must be warned in advance that the response to MUA is often disappointing in patients who have diabetes.

Arthroscopic or open surgical release

If MUA fails, it is possible to surgically cut through the coraco-humeral ligament producing an immediate improvement in the shoulder's range of movement.[3] This can be done through an arthroscope or through an open shoulder incision. In most cases this is immediately effective.

Outcome

Even in cases of frozen shoulder that are said to have 'resolved', Schaffer[4] has shown that over 50% of so-called 'resolved' cases have a long-term residual restriction of movement.

Rotator cuff disease

Rotator cuff disease is a spectrum of problems that range from impingement syndrome to full blown rotator cuff arthropathy. Most patients who develop rotator cuff disease are aged over 40 and most have problems on their dominant side. MRI scans on healthy volunteers reveal complete rotator cuff tears in about 14% of people and incomplete tears in 20%, indicating that it is possible to have near normal shoulder function despite substantial rotator cuff damage. Over the age of 60, 54% of people have a rotator cuff tear on MRI. It is clear that operative decisions should not be based solely on MRI evidence. The reasons for these findings are unknown, but it may be that the

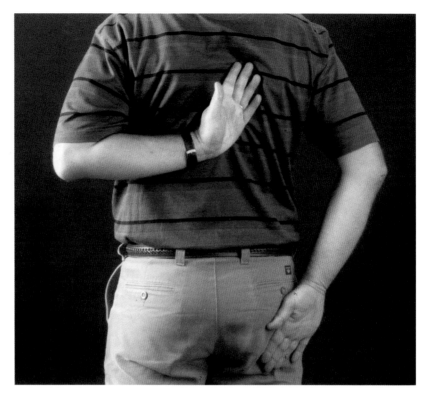

Figure 11.1
Frozen shoulder

Fifty-one year old patient recovering from a right-sided frozen shoulder. The patient is attempting to internally rotate his shoulder. On the affected side, he can only reach the level of his buttock, in contrast to the rotation achieved with the non-affected shoulder.

location of the tear is more important than size. The rotator cuff would also appear to have considerable reserve function.

Impingement

Impingement is the first stage in rotator cuff disease. Impingement is characterised by pain around the shoulder and down the muscles of the arm. There is usually a painful arc of movement. The arm can be abducted to 90 degrees before pain begins and if it gets past 120 degrees can be pain-free again. The patient may blame overhead or repetitive activities and pain is made worse by reaching or trying to put the hand behind the back. Typical problems are doing up a bra or tucking the back of a shirt into trousers. Hawkins sign is positive (see Figure 11.2). Muscle weakness or wasting is not normally present, but there may be pain on resisted movements. An injection of a small amount of 2% lignocaine into the subacromial space may completely obliterate the pain and stiffness within five minutes and confirms the diagnosis.

Any space-occupying lesion within the subacromial space may lead to impingement. This may be a bursitis, calcific deposits, the swollen edges of a cuff tear, or the presence of bony spurs. Ultrasound or MRI scanning may show changes within the rotator cuff.

Figure 11.2
Hawkins sign

This patient has subacromial impingement. This condition can be tested for by flexing the elbow to 90 degrees and rotating the patient's hand and forearm down from the shoulder.

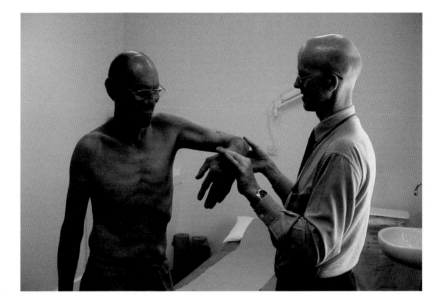

Treatment for impingement syndrome

Steroid injection with local anaesthetic into the subacromial space is effective in relieving pain and improving movement in the short term. The injection is aimed at the leading edge of the coraco–acromial ligament through an anterolateral or posterolateral approach. There may be a temporary exacerbation of symptoms afterwards. Physiotherapy aimed at the scapula muscles helps strengthen and rehabilitate a dysfunctional cuff.

Surgery, whether open or arthroscopic, involves resection of the anterior part of the acromion and usually division of the coraco-acromial ligament. It is indicated for longstanding symptoms not responding to conservative measures. Recovery is slow after surgery and supervised physiotherapy is usually necessary. However, the rate of recovery often depends on the motivation of the patient.

Rotator cuff tears

The shoulder is a fundamentally unstable joint. It is held in place by a group of structures referred to as the rotator cuff. The rotator cuff is made up of the tendons of supraspinatus, infraspinatus, subscapularis and teres minor, the joint capsule, and ligamentous reinforcements. The long head of the biceps is also involved. When the cuff tears, the stabilising effect on the humeral head is lost and this allows abnormal movements at the joint. Cuff tears are common and partial cuff tears often occur in young athletic patients. The incidence of tears increases with age.

Cause and classification

It's still not clear why rotator cuff tears occur. They may be caused by impingement or by injuries to the tendons. Cuff tears are classified as being partial or full thickness and by their size. Most tears are thought to begin in the supraspinatus tendon. There may be an acute, chronic, or acute-on-chronic presentation of pain, and often loss of power. In severe cases complete loss of active arm abduction occurs; the patient has to lift the arm up using the opposite hand and is unable to hold it there unaided. However, passive movements are usually maintained and this helps us to distinguish the condition from frozen shoulder.

Treatment of rotator cuff tears[6]

Treatment of rotator cuff tears in the under-70s is usually surgical. Small tears can be repaired via an open or arthroscopic route, usually combined with a subacromial decompression. Larger tears and more chronic tears, especially those in the elderly, are more difficult to repair. However, subacromial decompression will usually help control pain, even in the more advanced stages.

Rotator cuff arthropathy: the final stage in rotator cuff disease

Rotator cuff arthropathy is the last stage in the continuum of rotator cuff disease. Following a massive tear, the head of the humerus moves so abnormally that it gradually erodes the undersurface of the acromial arch.[7] This is readily diagnosed on plain X-rays, but treatment is difficult. It's now possible to treat rotator cuff arthropathy by replacing the shoulder,[8] but results are much poorer than those for glenohumeral arthritis. Special types of prosthesis have been designed to attempt to address this problem.

Tears of the biceps tendon

In some patients, the tendon of the biceps muscle ruptures. Biceps actually has three tendons, two of which insert around the shoulder (hence the name biceps). The third tendon inserts into the radius, just below the elbow. In most cases the proximal 'long head' ruptures and the bulk of the muscle flops down towards the elbow. This is sometimes referred to as the 'Popeye' sign as the patient has a new, bulging muscle mass in the lower part of their arm (see Figure 11.3). In these cases we usually rehabilitate the patient gradually with physiotherapy. Basically, the second ('short head') is still attached to the scapula and the remaining 'good' muscle fibres can hypertrophy although the lump in the lower half of the humerus doesn't go away. Rupture of the long head is more common in inflammatory conditions such as rheumatoid arthritis. Very occasionally, the distal head ruptures and the muscle belly springs upwards, creating an obvious mass at the top half of the arm. This is more debilitating and makes it difficult to turn a screw driver. In this situation, some surgeons would consider surgical repair.

Figure 11.3
Rupture of the long head of the biceps

The belly of the biceps muscle is prominent and has flopped down towards the elbow – the so-called 'Popeye' sign. It is usually treated conservatively.

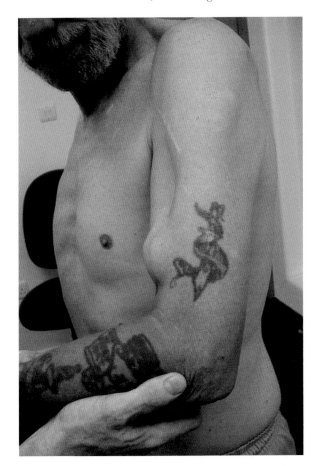

The dislocated shoulder

The shoulder is by far the most mobile joint in the human body. Unfortunately, this remarkable range of movement can only be achieved by sacrificing stability and the shoulder is also the most commonly dislocated joint. A dislocated shoulder should be reduced *promptly*. If a dislocated shoulder is left unreduced, the ligaments around it soon stretch and become ineffective. Between five and seven days post-injury, it becomes impossible to relocate the joint by closed methods. If there is any doubt about shoulder dislocation, do X-rays in two planes.

Who dislocates their shoulder?

There are two groups of patients who dislocate their shoulders:

1. young patients who receive high-energy injuries, such as rugby players
2. older people with weak rotator cuffs receiving low-energy injuries.

Almost all shoulder dislocations are **anterior**, with less than 5% being posterior. Posterior shoulder dislocations sometimes follow epileptic fits or electrocution.

In a typical scenario, when a young patient dislocates his/her shoulder for the first time it is usually an anterior dislocation resulting from a violent event. The patient will be able to give a clear-cut history of a dramatic injury during a contact sport or a fall. There is sudden swelling, immobility, and pain around the joint. When compared to the normal side, the shoulder usually looks 'dislocated'. The joint has to be relocated, usually under anaesthetic in the A&E department or in theatre. The arm is immobilised in a sling for three to four weeks and the patient is then referred to physiotherapy for active mobilisation. Some surgeons now advocate immobilising the arm in external rotation. This position is cumbersome but may reduce the risk of recurrence.

Recurrent dislocations

Paradoxically, the younger a patient is with a first-time dislocation, the more likely they are to have a recurrence. About one in three become recurrent dislocators. This means that they repeatedly present with a shoulder dislocation that needs reducing – often after trivial injuries. Eventually, there may be a subjective sense of subluxation or dislocation practically all the time.

Older adults, especially those over the age of 65, are more likely to be once-only dislocators. On the negative side, older adults are often left with a stiff shoulder after their dislocation.

Mechanisms of dislocation and investigations

As mentioned, shoulder dislocation almost always means anterior dislocation. These patients have often torn vital structures around the shoulder joint. In a classic 1938 paper, Bankart[9] described a common lesion in unstable shoulders – that the anterior part of the glenoid labrum is torn off allowing the head of the humerus to dislocate out of the front of the joint. At this moment, the back of the head may collide with the edge of the glenoid. This produces an indentation in the humeral head called a **Hill–Sachs lesion**, and this defect may be seen on an axillary view X-ray. The best way to assess the damage is by MRI scanning, sometimes with the addition of a contrast agent (MRI arthrography). This enables the torn labrum and any additional tears in the capsule to be seen.

Recurrent dislocation and other instabilities[10]

Recurrent shoulder dislocation is a significant disability and these patients can be offered surgery. By performing an MRI scan, the shoulder surgeon is now able to plan a repair operation for the individual patient's injury before they are admitted.

Although there are a variety of operations available, a number of standard terms crop up. The Bankart operation repairs the Bankart lesion and involves re-attaching the torn labrum into bone.[9] The Putti Platt operation involves reefing the subscapularis muscle. The Bristow Laterjet procedure attempts to move extra muscles in front of the shoulder to stop it dislocating.

It is now possible to perform stabilisation operations through an arthroscope, although many procedures still require open surgery.

Postoperative care

Postoperatively, the patient has to wear a shoulder immobiliser for six weeks before starting graduated physiotherapy exercises. They should not return to contact sports for at least six months. Even after final recovery from a shoulder repair, the range of movement may be restricted, especially external rotation. An undisciplined and unreliable patient is not a good candidate for shoulder surgery.

Posterior dislocations

These are rare, but when they do occur, they may be associated with specific accidents, such as epileptic fitting and electrocution. Because of their rarity and because they are difficult to see on an AP shoulder

X-ray, junior doctors often misdiagnose patients with posterior dislocation. In fact, 30% of these injuries are missed on initial assessment. Even a career shoulder surgeon will only see a modest number of posterior dislocations in his lifetime and there is a lack of consensus within the profession as to how to best treat posterior dislocations.

Multidirectional instability

Some patients develop a form of instability that is not specifically anterior or posterior but **multidirectional**. The shoulder tends to sublux with everyday activity. There is sometimes an association with generalised joint laxity. It is often treated effectively by physiotherapy, but surgery to tighten the capsule may be offered in refractory cases.

Voluntary dislocation

Voluntary, or habitual, dislocators are rare but do exist. Some school children develop an ability to dislocate the shoulder at will and often use it as an excuse to escape from lessons. The crucial observation to make in these children is that the act of dislocation is not painful. Surgery should be avoided!

Shoulder osteoarthritis and replacement surgery

Glenohumeral osteoarthritis is associated with true shoulder pain; i.e. anterior and lateral pain over the shoulder itself. The shoulder is not a weight-bearing joint and OA here is much less common than in the hip or knee.

Shoulder osteoarthritis shows up well on a plain X-ray, with classical features of decreased glenohumeral joint space, sclerosis, marginal osteophytes, and cysts. On examination, rough crepitus is often felt in the joint. There may be an effusion. Surgery is rarely necessary except in the most painful cases.

Acromioclavicular osteoarthritis is more common and presents with pain and tenderness that is well-localised over the acromioclavicular joint, often with associated swelling. Arm adduction across the chest can be painful. Excision of the distal end of the clavicle may be carried out in such patients, usually to good effect.

Rheumatoid arthritis

In mono-articular RA the shoulder may be affected in isolation, but it may also be part of a generalised rheumatoid picture. RA begins with the process of synovial inflammation and this is followed by degenerative change in the glenohumeral joint itself. Patients are often referred to the orthopaedic surgeon by their rheumatologist. In other words, by the time they see an orthopaedic surgeon the disease may be well advanced.

Shoulder replacement[11]

At first sight, a shoulder replacement looks like the upper limb equivalent of a hip replacement. However, experience with shoulder replacements is far less extensive than with hips and the results can be disappointing. The operation often eliminates pain. The range of movement may be improved after shoulder replacement, but it is unlikely to go back to normal. The main indication for shoulder replacement is unremitting pain, especially from OA. It may also be considered after comminuted fractures of the proximal humerus and in RA. A patient with a stiff painless shoulder is unlikely to benefit from a shoulder replacement.

Elbow problems

Tennis elbow affects the common extensor origin at the lateral epicondyle. **Golfer's elbow** affects the common flexor origin at the medial epicondyle. A number of muscles take origin from these prominences. Degenerative changes at either of these sites can cause pain and tenderness over the elbow, termed 'epicondylitis'. They are often associated with over-use activities such as racquet sports. Although the name suggests an inflammatory cause, histology of the affected tissue reveals degenerative changes and often represents a chronic injury/reparative cycle.

Lateral epicondylitis[12]

Tennis elbow is nine times more common than golfer's elbow and is caused by over-use activities, classically playing the backhand in tennis. It tends to affect the dominant elbow and is most common in the fourth decade of life. If the pain radiates down the forearm, consider the possibility of involvement of the posterior interosseous nerve. The main tests are the detection of tenderness over the lateral epicondyle and pain on resisted extension of the middle finger. There is also pain when trying to lift up a chair with outstretched hands.

Medial epicondylitis

Golfer's elbow is much less common than lateral epicondylitis and tends to occur in the non-dominant elbow. There may be an associated ulnar nerve entrapment with paraesthesiae in the little finger and medial aspect of the palm.

Treatment for tennis and golfer's elbow

Just about any treatment works, since 90% of cases resolve within six to 12 months, during which time the symptoms may wax and wane. Active treatments include ultrasound, physiotherapy, splints, and steroid injections. Topical NSAIDs appear to be effective for short-term pain relief. Less convincing treatments include acupuncture and the intake of vitamins. Surgical treatment can be offered to the 10% that do not resolve within 12 months. This involves excising an ellipse of degenerative tissue from the tender area.

Osteoarthritis of the elbow

Primary OA of the elbow is rare. It can occur following the repetitive lifting of heavy loads, such as that experienced by weight lifters or heavy manual workers. There is pain when the elbow is fully extended. Carrying even a relatively light item such as a briefcase with the elbow fully extended may be very painful. Paradoxically, some patients develop significant stiffness and little in the way of pain.

Loose bodies in the elbow

Loose bodies result from osteochondritis dissecans, or acute or repetitive trauma, or may be idiopathic. Loose pieces of cartilage may actually grow in size once trapped within the joint. They may cause joint snapping, locking, or catching. Surgical removal can be performed arthroscopically or through an open procedure. Results are usually excellent, unless there is associated painful osteoarthritis.

Ulnar nerve entrapment at the elbow

The ulnar nerve is affected by entrapment neuropathy where it passes behind the medial epicondyle. This is the second most common entrapment neuropathy after carpal tunnel syndrome and the two may coexist. Patients often describe a burning or aching pain in the little and ring fingers. Symptoms are made worse by fully flexing the elbows or resting the elbows on a hard surface. There is usually a positive Tinel's sign over the nerve at the elbow, just behind the medial epicondyle. In severe cases where there is motor involvement the small muscles of the hand may be wasted and this is usually irreversible, even once the entrapment has been decompressed. The results of surgery are less pre-dictable than those for carpal tunnel syndrome.

Brachial plexus injuries[13]

The classical mechanism of injury is that of a motorcyclist hitting the ground, shoulder first. The head is pushed away from the shoulder abruptly and the nerve roots to the brachial plexus snap or are severely damaged.

A complete brachial plexus injury results in flail limb. This is a com-pletely 'dead' arm, with no motor or sensory function at all. Ulti-mately, some patients may even request amputation, because the arm serves no function and simply gets in the way.

If the injury is a neuropraxia, with the nerves traumatised but still intact, then some function may return over a period of many months. If there has been no return of function at 12 months, it is likely that the deficit will be permanent. The extent of disability will depend on which nerves have been affected and at what level. Early exploration and repair is sometimes performed within the first six weeks.

Peripheral nerves grow at the rate of about 1mm a day once recovery has begun, so at best they will grow 36.5cm in a year. A brachial plexus injury is a long way from the fingers, so recovery is unpredictable. For a peripheral nerve to regenerate as far as the hand following a nerve root injury is difficult, and by the time it eventually gets there, many of the specialised receptor cell bodies will have shut down and died off because they have had no nerve supply. Many attempts to surgically correct a flail limb have been made over the years, some of them highly imaginative, but none uniformly successful. The group with the most cause for optimism is children, who have better powers of recovery and shorter arms. Any procedure to help this devastating injury is best attempted in one of the few specialist centres in the country.

References

1. Codman EA. Tendinitis of the short rotators. In: Codman EA [ed]. *The Shoulder: rupture of the supraspinatus tendon and other lesions in or about the subacromial bursa.* Boston, MA: Thomas Todd and Co, 1934.

2. Bunker TD, Anthony PP. The pathology of frozen shoulder: a Dupuytren-like dis-ease. *J Bone Joint Surg Am* 1995; **77B:** 677–83.

3. Chambler A F, Carr A J. The role of surgery in frozen shoulder. *J Bone Joint Surg Br* 2003; **85(6):** 789–95.

4. Schaffer B, Tibone JE, Kerlan RK. Frozen shoulder: a long term follow up. *J Bone Joint Surg Am* 1992; **74A:** 738–46.

5. Solomon L, Warwick D, Nayagam S. The shoulder and pectoral guide. In: *Apley's System of Orthopaedics and Fractures.* [8th edition] New York: OUP-USA, 2001.

6. Severud EL, Ruotolo C, Abbott D, Nottage WM. All arthroscopic versus mini open repair. A long term retrospective outcome comparison. *Arthroscopy* 2003; **(3):** 234–8.

7. Feeney MS, O'Dowd J, Kay EW, Colville J. Glenohumeral articular cartilage changes in rotator cuff disease. *J Shoulder Elbow Surg* 2003; **1:** 20–3.

8. Sarris IK, Papadimitriou NG, Sotereanaes DG. Bipolar hemiarthroplasty for chronic rotator cuff tear arthropathy. *J Arthroplasty* 2003; **2:** 169–73.

9. Bankart ASB. The pathology and treatment of recurrent dislocation of the shoulder-joint. *Brit J Surg* 1938; **26:** 23–29.

10. Gill TJ, Zarins B. Open repairs for the treatment of anterior shoulder instability. *Am J Sports Med* 2003; **31(1):** 142–53.

11. Iannotti JP, Norris TR. Influence of preoperative factors on outcome of shoulder arthroplasty for glenohumeral osteoarthritis. *J Bone Joint Surg Am* 2003; **85-A(2):** 251–8.

12. Assendelft W, Green S, Buchbinder R, *et al.* Tennis elbow. *BMJ* 2003; **327:** 329–30.

13. Birch R. Brachial plexus injuries. *J Bone Joint Surgery Am* 1996; **78B:** 986–92.

Index